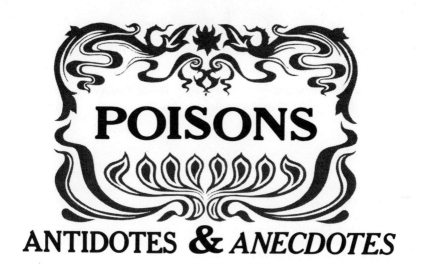

POISONS

ANTIDOTES & ANECDOTES

BY WILLIAM TICHY

 STERLING PUBLISHING CO., INC. NEW YORK

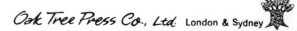 Oak Tree Press Co., Ltd. London & Sydney

OTHER BOOKS OF INTEREST

Butter Side Up
It's An Odd World
The Curious Book
Nature at Its Strangest

Oddball Fishes
Strangely Enough
Weirdest People in the World
Would You Believe . . . ?

Would You Believe This, Too?

The author and publishers wish to thank the following individuals and organizations for their contributions of illustrations and information: A. Abei, Director, Federal Poisons Office, Switzerland; British Information Services, London; John J. Crotty, Director, National Clearinghouse for Poison Control Centers, U.S.; Roy Goulding, Director, National Poisons Information Service, U.K.; Lawrence A. Heimlich, B-D Life Support Systems; Kenneth E. Lucas, California Academy of Sciences; R. C. McCarthy, Senior Pharmaceutical Inspector, Dept. of Public Health, S. Austral.; J. Ross, Senior Poisons Control Officer, Dept. of Public Health, Austral.; E. H. W. Shepard, Dept. of Health and Social Security London; U.S. Fish and Wildlife Service; A. N. P. van Heijst, Dutch National Poison Information Centre; G. N. Volans, Deputy Director, National Poisons Information Service, U.K.

Cover by Guy Brison-Stack

Copyright © 1977 by Sterling Publishing Co., Inc.
419 Park Avenue South, New York, N.Y. 10016
Distributed in Australia and New Zealand by Oak Tree Press Co., Ltd.,
P.O. Box J34, Brickfield Hill, Sydney 2000, N.S.W.
Distributed in the United Kingdom and elsewhere in the British Commonwealth
by Ward Lock Ltd., 116 Baker Street, London W 1
Manufactured in the United States of America
All rights reserved
Library of Congress Catalog Card No.:76-51188

Sterling ISBN 0-8069-3738-6 Trade   Oak Tree 7061-2553-3
3739-4 Library

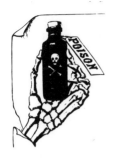

Contents

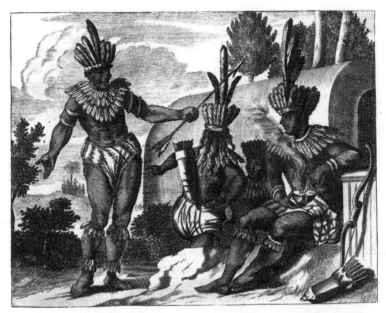

The Peruvian Indians maintained an arsenal of poison-tipped arrows.

Poison Fundamentals

Simple question: "What is a poison?" Simple answer? No, there have been arguments over a poison definition for many years. When does a substance which can be a useful medicine become a deadly poison? And what happens when the question goes to court?

These are only a few modern twists to the centuries-old problem of poisons.

Introduction

Primitive people knew of poisons eons ago. They worshipped poisonous plants, attributing their lethal power to the supernatural and the occult. Demons, they feared, lived in the roots of plants and when disturbed or displeased they arose and drove the violators to madness and delirium. Ancient Greeks and Romans believed that the lowly mushroom sprang from a bolt of night lightning, and that the venom of poisonous animals caused intoxication.

It seems only natural that before there was a scientific way of looking at the poisonous plants, animals and noxious materials of the earth there would be a more humble way of looking at these potent forces. There was, and it was the thoroughly human approach called folklore, where all the knowledge of a popular and intriguing subject is found in the form of stories and traditional tales.

Nearly all the deadly poisons and maladies of man had a remedy in folklore, and antidotes came to outnumber the poisons and maladies themselves by a fantastic number. This isn't too surprising, considering that the number of poisons is at least roughly limited by nature while the antidotes of folklore were limited mostly by the imagination. The same poison would lead to a different antidote in India from the one devised, perhaps, by the ancient Persians. Consider a quick sampling of antidotes of different places and different times. There's the old Scottish antidote for deafness: take ant's eggs, mix them with the juice of onions, and drop them deftly in the ear. There's a tropical antidote for the chills of malaria: put a large live spider in a bag and wear it around the neck. The bezoar stone of colonial America had broad powers. It was good against the bite of mad dogs, scorpions, and all other venomous animals. It was so valuable that it took a whole community to afford just one. The gold wedding ring was the old antidote for warts and sties. Amulets, talismans, and magic potions were all associated with some mystical power, and the more universally potent the object, the more it was sought after.

Today much of the world still believes in the superstition and lore of poisons and antidotes, as if the science of poisons didn't even exist. Progress has been phenomenal in scientific achievement, but knowledge about poisons is more secretive than ever. There's super-biological warfare with enough of SATANS virus to depopulate half the world, and there's the assassin's variety that is aimed at only one target. In both cases the object is to bring toxicity to some new peak of power.

Consider for just a moment this exchange between James Bond, Agent 007, and his boss in Ian Fleming's *Dr. No*. " 'By the way, did you ever discover what the stuff was that Russian woman put into him?' 'Got the answer yesterday. . . . Taken us three months. It was a bright chap at the School of Tropical Medicine who came up with it. The drug was fugu poison. The Japanese use it for committing suicide. It comes from the sex organs of the Japanese globe-fish. Trust the Russians to use something no one's even heard of. They might as well have used curare. It has much the same effect—paralysis of the central nervous system. Fugu's scientific name is Tetrodoxin. It's terrible stuff and very quick. One shot of it like your man got and in a matter of seconds the motor and respiratory muscles are paralysed. At first the chap sees double and then he can't keep his eyes open. Next he can't swallow. His head falls and he can't raise it. Dies of respiratory paralysis.' "* (The tetrodoxin mentioned has 100,000 times the numbing power of a medical anesthetic. Later on we'll discuss a dangerous delicacy, fugu stew, recommended for only the most courageous gourmets.)

The Central Intelligence Agency of the United States has weaponry that could shake the Rock of Gibraltar. The CIA calls it "007 hardware." Included are dart guns that shoot minuscule poison darts the length of a football field into the victim, where they promptly dissolve and vanish without leaving a trace. There are other dart guns too; some that look like an umbrella or a fountain pen, another that looks like an ordinary walking stick. There's also the fluorescent lamp that gives off a poisonous gas when turned on, and a heat-sensitive engine bolt that gives off a poisonous gas when the car starts. One of the most exotic poisons of all is contained in a simple button which can be worn secretly across borders or into forbidden places.

All of this brings up a question which has plagued many a curious youngster: "Why does it take so little poison to kill a full-grown man?" How do we explain the fact that poison like Dr. No's fugu poison demolishes a man weighing 500 million times as much as the deadly dose! Part of this book is dedicated to the answer.

There is enormous value in knowing exactly what to do in the event of your own or someone else's poisoning. Each year there are a million cases of poisoning in the world, and more than 15,000 deaths. An alarming number of these victims are children under the age of five. The Poison Control Centers

*Ian Fleming, *Dr. No*, © 1958, Macmillan, Inc.

around the world are at war against death by poison. This war against poison is reported, the current situation considered and summaries of poisons, antidotes, treatment and instant action presented to serve as your guide to poison prevention.

Overall, this book will introduce you to the romance and intrigue of poisons and antidotes, presenting facts, fundamentals and a modern point of view. We will explore the world of *deadly* poisons—cobra venom, not poison ivy—since the substances which claim their victims permanently have always held the greatest fascination. Here you will discover some of the truly exotic poisons of nature, and learn the proper action to take against poison emergencies, whether common or exotic.

Poisons Defined

Sir Robert Christison, the famous 19th century toxicologist, once wrote: "What then is a poison? Some will have settled outright for a definition. But although the most skillful have tried to define a poison, everyone has hitherto failed." This was written over a hundred years ago, but "poison" is still a hard word to define today. What's the problem? A good definition is one that means the same thing all the time. Consider the case of morphine, a beneficial drug. In small doses it relieves pain and relaxes the body. In larger amounts it is deadly. Exactly when did it turn from a beneficial substance into a poison? Lead, like several other minerals, gradually builds up in the body. Each small daily dose in itself may be handled as if it were harmless, but as with the "straw that broke the camel's back" there's one dose that kills. Copper in small doses is vital. In doses slightly too large it poisons the heart muscle. Fluoride in small doses hardens tooth enamel, yet one teaspoonful (5 grams) taken at one time will kill. In a sense even candy is deadly. Suppose it leads to overweight? Insurance company tables will prove that it kills: their weight versus years of life charts show fewer years of life for plumper persons. In this light candy is a poison. We can see that saying what is or what is not a poison just . . . depends.

COURTROOM CONTROVERSY

When it comes to the law the simple question "What is a poison?" takes on the tension of courtroom drama. A Scotland Yard scientist and former director of New York's Metropolitan Police Laboratory sees the question in the light of the law: "The difficulty of defining a poison is unimportant in everyday life, where no one says 'pass the strychnine, please'—but it is anathema to the law, for which black should be black and white white, with never the twain overlapping. The law gets around that difficulty quite simply by not trying to define a poison. It merely specifies by name the various substances that are to be deemed poisons for its purpose; hence the various lists and schedules under the Poisons Acts. Even this, however, is not enough. A good many years ago I had to analyze a cup of Ovaltine or Horlick's or some such drink which had been turned in to the police by an aggrieved Bristol wife. It appeared that her husband thought her too tense and excitable, and had tried to calm her down by putting some barbiturate sleeping tablets in the drink, unknown to her. It was by no means an excessive amount—in fact, just about the right dosage for this purpose—but she took exception to being so treated without her consent, as most of us would. So he was prosecuted for administering a 'noxious' substance to his wife. The defense was that the amount of barbiturate given could do her no harm, therefore it was not a 'noxious' substance. The prosecution relied on me as a witness to say that it was. I said, which seemed to me sufficient to my simple unlegalistic mind, that a barbiturate was by definition noxious, because it was named as a poison on schedules 1 and 4 of the Pharmacy and Poisons Act of 1939. However, the magistrates were unimpressed by this argument and the husband was acquitted. . . ."*

In brief: As a compromise we define a poison as any compound which in relatively small quantities and by its chemical actions can cause death or disability.

Antidotes Defined

Poisons and antidotes go together like hand and glove. The Spaniards, when they explored South America for the first time, for example, were poisoned by the curare carried on the tips of the Indian arrows. Their answer was to apply the juice of garlic to the wound. This was their working antidote. A favorite antidote for snakebite, popular in the United States between 1830 and 1870, was whiskey (the old moonshiner expression "a shot of snakebite" probably refers to this favored antidote). The European answer to snakebite was an antidote of strong wine and hot pepper. Modern medicine answers with the antivenin for snakebite . . . and offers a long list of other compounds that dull the actions of poison as well.

In brief: An antidote is any substance that nulls the effects of a poison on the spot and prevents its absorption, or blocks its destructive action once absorbed.

*H. J. Walls, *Scotland Yard Scientist: My Thirty Years in Forensic Science*, Taplinger Publishing Co., © 1972 by H. J. Walls.

Poison Mysteries and
Madness Through the Ages

Poisons have always held a peculiar fascination for mankind, as shown by the unceasing efforts to control these potent substances for hunting and warfare, and the innumerable antidotes, amulets, talismans, fetishes and charms conjured up to protect against their deadly power throughout history.

Primitive tribes provide us with a true "window into the past." We have good reason to believe that their whims and ways have changed little over the ages. We see them as "pros" at hunting and fishing with the tools of poison, whether stupefying fish and scooping them off the surface of the water like so much driftwood, or felling bird and beast with minuscule poison darts. And in the Renaissance we see another generation of "pros," but now in the guise of "Poison Cults" and "Super-amateurs"—like the Borgias and Madame de Brinvilliers—who, as we shall see, committed atrocities so horrible that they can hardly be believed.

In the Beginning

A long, long time ago there was an unknown tribesman who picked a poison berry . . . and suffered the worst for it. That's when our knowledge of poisons began. From that time—whenever it was—our knowledge grew and was passed down through countless generations, by word of mouth or contained in tribal rituals. Soon it became too much for ordinary tribesmen, and medicine men took the reins.

They made man's knowledge of poisons grow even faster but kept it within secret circles, away from ordinary members of the tribe. It was intended only for the witchdoctor, the chief, his family and a few of the chosen. From the time of the witchdoctors' takeover knowledge of poisons always remained under the control of a small group of people.

The art of poisoning developed as a means to extend man's power to kill, both animals for food and his fellow man in battle. As early as 1700 B.C. the Scythians used poisons mixed with human blood on their arrows. The European nomads also used poisoned arrowheads. Aristotle tells of their use by the Celts, a warlike peoples who defeated the Roman army in 390 B.C. Poisons as a special kind of weapon appeal to man's baser instincts because

- they are silent, leaving no blood or signs of violence
- they make deception extremely easy
- they are inexpensive and usually available
- they can be used to eliminate individuals or entire armies.

Wily commanders such as Julius Caesar have been known to feign retreat, "accidentally" leaving behind casks of wine spiked with stupefying drugs. They allowed the "victors" to drink and celebrate, then, when the "victors" were sleeping it off, returned and wiped out the whole enemy army.

The Special Role of Mythology

The first solid evidence that man had thoughts and feelings about poisons was in mythology. At the very beginning of recorded history, in Babylonia at about 4500 B.C., there was a goddess of poisons called Gulla. Her various names suggest a little about her: "Terrible Goddess," "Mistress of Charms and Spells" and "Controller of Noxious Poisons." Little else is known about her. Then centuries later came Hecate, the Greek goddess of witchcraft, the caster of spells, the founder of sorcery and the first to discover the existence of poisonous plants. Following her came Circe, one of the first of the Great Sorceresses, well portrayed in Homer's famous tale, the *Odyssey*.

Circe was the witch goddess who lived in the land of Aeaea. She was so beautiful that no man could resist her. With this charm she lured travellers—usually lonely sailors —to stay on her island and drink from her enchanted cup. With one swallow the strangers turned into swine and were driven to the goddess's great sty. There they would remain forever, living with the mind they had when human but now entrapped in the body of an ordinary looking hog. When Homer's hero, Odysseus, arrived in Aeaea his crew was promptly drawn into Circe's spell and turned into swine —all but one. Odysseus himself escaped by the magic of an herb given him by Hermes, the god of herbs, commerce, and travel and messenger to all the gods. The magic herb (the first antidote?) made him immune to her magic spell.

Poisons of the Primitive Tribes

The use of poison by man reaches back into time even farther than mythology, to the beginning of man's struggle with nature, in fact, but besides a few artifacts found in the gravesites of early man from about 50,000 years ago, we have little knowledge of primitive man's way of life. Unless, that is, we look at the life styles of modern primitives and assume that what we have is really a "window on the past." Anthropologists studying primitive races find that what they see today reflects the way men lived hundreds or thousands of years ago. Bows and arrows are used just as in the Stone Age, and it is safe to assume their use of poisons hasn't changed much either. The first and most important use of poisons was help in the hunt. Often it was poison darts, arrows and spears that made success in the hunt, and therefore survival, possible.

TRIBES OF AFRICA

The Bushmen of South Africa are confined to a very desolate region known as the Kalahari Desert, but somehow they have managed to discover several formidable poisons. Witnesses tell of victims dying slowly and in great agony, giving out finally in a surge of violent delirium. This poison comes from the entrails of a small native caterpillar. Arrows are "double dipped" for use against lions, giraffes and other large animals. More common poisons are extracted from scorpions, spiders, and puff-adders. (The puff-adder is a large sluggish snake which gets its name from the fact that it "puffs" out its breath.)

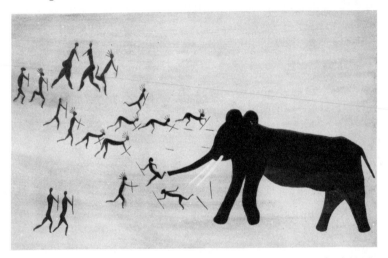

Bushman hunters use poisoned spears to hunt a massive elephant in this cave painting from South Africa.

The Pygmies of Central Africa happen to be the smallest humans on earth, averaging 4 feet 11 inches, but the effect of their favorite arrow poison is anything but diminutive. Derived from the formidable red ant, it is so poisonous that a single poisoned arrow will fell a full-grown elephant.

In West Africa there are several tribes which use poisons for hunting—*and* to preserve tribal law and order by the "ordeal of poison." They use a poison called "mauvi" in their trial-by-ordeal rituals. Mauvi is made by scraping the bark from a certain tree—known only to the witchdoctor—and mixing it with water.

The rites of the ordeal are very specific. The brew is given to both the one accused of wrongdoing and his accuser. The natives believe that the guilty one will die. If the brew is good, death will be quick: vomiting, convulsions, then death, rapidly and in that order. If it turns out that both parties merely throw up and live, then the brew is declared "badly prepared" and the contest is, so to speak, temporarily a draw—temporarily because a new brew is prepared and the contest continues until death actually points its ghastly finger at the wrongdoer. When death does finally occur the guilty one's wife and children are also put to death. All terms of the tribal contract are carried out and overseen by a highly rewarded tribal official who must also pay the brewers' fee. The natives believe this test is infallible and submit to it eagerly to prove their innocence if they are ever accused of evil deeds.

THE ARUNTA OF AUSTRALIA

The Arunta are a wandering tribe of the Australian desert. They too are among the most primitive peoples on earth. Stone knives, spears, and other archaic implements are used just as they were in the Stone Age with one possible exception: their boomerang, which would be too modern for Stone Age man. They hunt with the spear when necessary but prefer an easier, sure-fire technique—the hunt by poison. After reaching a water hole the tribesmen drink as much as they can, then poison the water with an extract of the pituri plant (*Duboisia hopwoodi* is the botanical name). Following this they wait for the thirsty regular visitors to drink the poisoned water. The most prized victim is the emu, an enormous ostrich-like bird, which the Arunta claim becomes paralyzed and drops before it gets 200 yards (180 metres) from the hole—nor do other animals fare better.

THE MALAY POISONERS

Malayans are experts with the blow dart. Novelist James A. Michener describes how they use and make their near perfect blow guns.

"I saw one of the strange weapons. They are extremely lethal and effective at distances up to two hundred feet [60 metres], for their tiny dart-like arrows are tipped with the dried gum of the ipoh tree, one of the most instantaneous jungle poisons known. During the emergency, communists tried to take over one long house (storage house for guns) as a center for operations, but the two reds were struck with darts from blowguns. The first dropped dead after two steps. The second ran screaming for a hundred yards [90 metres] and died.

The blowgun I saw was about eight feet [240 centimetres] long and was made possible only because the jungle north of Kuala Lumpur produces a unique bamboo that has between its nodes a smooth, absolutely straight stretch of eight or nine feet [240 or 270 centimetres]. Such length, if cleaned out carefully inside, is as true and as strong as a rifle barrel, but for protection is housed inside a second, and slightly larger, length of bamboo. A mouthpiece is attached, and darts are made of palm fiber, light, true and very sharp. Tipped with ipoh poison, a dart is slipped into the interior bamboo barrel and the blowgun is raised to the lips. With a sudden burst of air from the lungs, the perfectly fitted dart is projected from the gun with considerable force. As we have seen, it can kill a man instantly. Eight or ten darts can kill a tiger. And there are even records of elephants having been brought down."*

It could even be said that the Malayans have a poison technology. The "long houses" have rows of differently colored darts, one color for each type of prospective game and one for

*James A. Michener, *Michener Miscellany, 1950–1970*, ©1973, Random House, Inc.

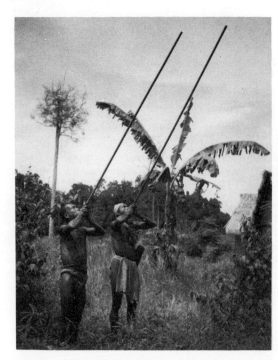

Two Malayan
hunters of the Sakai
tribe aim their
blowguns.

each concentration of poison. They are well aware that poisons are often "selective": that is, what is poisonous for one kind of game is not poisonous for another. Opium, for instance, is poisonous to man but not to pigeons. Hemlock is poisonous to man, but not goats, and henbane, deadly to fowl, is the rabbit's favorite food. The blue darts, for example, have just the right poison for one of the popular Malayan game birds.

In Java and Borneo, in what is known as the Eastern Archipelago, the natives have another very effective dart poison made from the sap of the upas tree and made into a super heart poison by adding the venom of scorpions and snakes. The upas is the legendary Poison Tree of Java. Stories circulated in Europe by world travelers stated that it was so poisonous that its

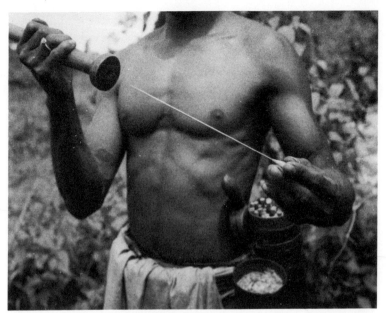
Inserting a poison dart into the barrel of a blowgun.

mere exhalations were fatal to all life—animal or vegetable—
for miles around and that its poison was collected by having
condemned criminals climb it. (Should they by some very slim
chance survive they were given full pardon.) The truth is that
the upas tree (botanically dubbed *Antiaris toxicaria*) does indeed
give off a powerful poison but nothing capable of destroying
life for miles around. A speck of the poison the size of a droplet
of mist is enough to kill a frog and an arrow prepared by the
Malayan recipe will kill a large animal in half an hour.

To prepare poison darts from the sap of the upas tree, it is
collected, put into a vessel fashioned out of palm trees and
cooked gently as it hangs safely above an open fire. After several
hours it becomes a viscous mass, in which condition it is rolled

up into palm leaves, tied at both ends with rattan and allowed to harden in this fashion. The hardened stick of poison is stored in this way until needed. Then some is scraped off, pulverized, mixed into a paste with water, smeared onto the dart tips, and the tips held near the fire and dried. Fire dries the poison into the wood and the dart is ready for use.

THE INDIANS OF CALIFORNIA

The Indians of California also used the poisoned water hole trick, but to catch fish rather than emus. They used a plant called soaproot (*Chlorogalum pomeridianum*) which they pulped, crushed, then dropped into a small body of water. Fish became stupefied and rose to the top, where the eager natives scooped them up by hand.

THE TAHITIANS

Natives of Tahiti first crush the fibrous wood of the narcotic plant *Hora papua* by beating it with a stick. Then, holding the bruised plant out of the water, they swim about, searching for the sight of a fish. Locating the fish they quickly dive down and anchor the poisonous plant under a rock or whatever is convenient at the moment. They repeat this operation several times, then return to the original location. If luck is with them, what they find is a handsome red mullet that looks dead. Only it isn't—it's merely paralyzed by the milky juices of *Hora papua*. As they are caught the fish are tossed into a canoe where, as one native put it: "By the time they wake up they will be dead."

THE SAMOANS

The Samoans are fishermen on a grand scale. They carefully place the pulverized kernels of the futu plant (*Barringtonia asiatica*) into reef holes and have divers take it into *deep* waters, where the catch is bigger but the effects are the same: stupefied fish rise helplessly to the surface.

THE PERUVIAN INDIANS

The Peruvian Indians have been known to use the peeled berries of a certain plant to stupefy a catch of fish. The only difference, perhaps, is that they are in the habit of watching the fish eat the berries, just before they conveniently rise to the surface. The poison in this instance is called picrotoxin.

THE AZTECS

Aztec Indians poisoned their fish with the root of the amolli plant (*Sapindus saponarius*).

THE HUMBOLDTS OF SOUTH AMERICA

The Humboldts use a plant known botanically as *Galega piscatorium* to make a sort of barbasco syrup with which to intoxicate fish and make them easy to catch by hand.

THE HAIRY AINUS

The Hairy Ainus of northern Japan are often called the white aborigines of Eastern Asia. They're a strange white race surrounded by yellow races, living a frigid existence, like the Eskimos of North America. And like the Eskimos they survive by whaling, but whaling with harpoons poisoned with deadly aconite. Whalers make a paste of the root called *Aconitum japanicum* by grinding it between two stones and mixing it with water. The paste is dried onto the harpoon, which is extremely effective, provided that the chief harpooner can navigate to within 50 feet (15 metres) of the target whale. Once hit, however, the whale surfaces for its last time in a few hours. Aconite is powerful enough to drop a smaller beast, like the bear, before it can run 100 yards (90 metres).

THE JIVAROS

The Jivaro Indians became famous for the plant known as barbasco. From this they prepare a poison to intoxicate fish; then, when totally "irrational," the fish are easily caught.

Fishing the Jivaro way requires a great deal of preparation as well as team work. One team piles rocks up in the stream to channel the fish into a small opening. Another team has the prepared root of the barbasco ready at the water's edge for the dawn after the barricade is put in place. (The root is pulverized until the poisonous juices ooze out.) Then promptly at the break of dawn the natives upstream put the prepared roots into the water and do a ritual dance. In an hour or so, after the poison begins to take effect, the fish suddenly begin to leap out of the water and gyrate crazily. The Jivaros now plunge into the water and the whole narrowed-down portion of the stream becomes alive with warriors, laughing and screaming with the greatest of joy, wrestling about for half-crazed fish.

The Lore of the Antidote

Antidotes, amulets, talismans, fetishes, charms and potions are names for the many and varied remedies conjured up by the wild imaginings of a desperate human race, made desperate by the stark realities of everyday existence. These words are used almost interchangeably in ordinary conversation, but there are a few subtle differences. "Antidote" includes all of the others: it is any remedy to counteract the effects of a poison. "Amulet" and "talisman," though now one and the same, were originally quite different. A talisman was a symbol engraved into stone or metal, or written on parchment or paper which served not only to ward off evils and poisons, but to produce love and affection in the beholder. The amulet was of much lower rank, since it was limited to poisons and other evils. Fetishes were also used to protect the owner, but they were not regarded as 100 per cent effective. Charms, on the other hand, always worked, usually relying on spells and witchcraft for their power. A potion is strictly a liquid medicine, available in different forms to cure both physical and emotional problems.

A glimpse into the remote past will explain why magical antidotes were needed. The first man lived in the vast forests of primeval days. He spent the entire day hunting for leaves, roots, and berries, stole eggs from angry birds, or killed a sparrow or a rabbit. When night came terror struck. He hid his wife and children behind huge boulders or in hollow trees, or in the shelter of caves from the ferocious animals who prowled about looking for something to feed to *their* mates or offspring.

Primitive man knew of poisons from his own daily experience. He thought that demons lived in the roots of plants and, when disturbed or displeased, these demons would take revenge by inflicting madness, delirium or death on the offender. As far as he could tell the demons were easily aroused, since everywhere he looked his comrades were dying of mysterious causes. What is understandable to the modern mind, familiar with the variety of poisonous nuts, berries, mushrooms and plants and the necessity for proper food preparation, was terrifying to our ignorant forefathers.

So primitive man felt a deep need for something with spiritual powers to protect him from the beasts and the demons. Amulets and talismans were such divinely endowed objects. The first amulets and talismans had three main missions: to get the "demon" out of the afflicted person, to ward off evils, and to sway other Spirits to do favors. These first primeval amulets were simple things: necklaces or pendants of bear's claws or oddly shaped rocks, perhaps blood red or purple. Then as time went on the complexity of the amulets increased. They became more like ornate jewelry and, at the same time, became associated with a ritual. Each disease required not only the right amulet but the right ritual, the words and actions to go with that amulet. At first ordinary men could manage but soon it required the services of a specialist. This was the origin of the witchdoctor, medicine man, shaman and priest.

Amulets and talismans were, and are, universal. They have always belonged to all peoples, all races, and over the countless centuries have taken on all of the art forms known to man. It's true that some will snicker at the weird claims and outlandish creations which follow—but it is well to remember that to tens of millions now living and millions upon millions long dead these claims and creations—their antidotes—were a big part of their *real* world.

Magically Endowed Stones

Mineral Stones: common, semi-precious and precious

Stone worship is as old as the art of talking to trees. Both reach back to the beginning when pebbles were worn as pendants or kept in caves for keepsakes. They flourished through the centuries until, when we reach the Middle Ages, we find as the only big seller in the apothecary shops . . . Medicine Rocks! The scene is much the same today, when Pet Rocks are given love and companionship. Rocks, it appears, were not always sought after because they were ornamental or could cure ills as medicine rocks, but rather because they were endowed with Spirits or personalities.

Even more, some rocks had supernatural powers! Rocks could be healthy or ill, grow old and die, move about and even transform themselves into wild beasts, should the occasion call for it. The Central American Indians, for instance, showed a great deal of respect for a huge rock that stood on top of a nearby mountain. The rock was shaped like a jaguar and could actually turn into one. Even the sages of ancient Greece were fanatic about rocks. They held that rocks could move about, make love and beget little rocks. And a few even maintained that the entire human race sprang from rocks. Pliny, the most famous scholar of first century Rome, wrote that rocks could heal and hypnotize. And he noted that some rocks had two sexes. The male sapphire, "as blue as the Mediterranean Sea," was darker than the female and had significantly greater power to hypnotize and heal. Another was the beautiful red ruby. Both sexes, conceded Pliny, had the ability to neutralize poisons but the male had far greater powers than the female.

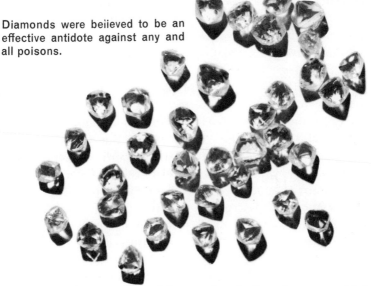

Diamonds were believed to be an effective antidote against any and all poisons.

Most of the stones used in amulets before (very roughly) 400 B.C. were semi-precious ones: the onyx, granite, moonstone, opal, jasper, amethyst, quartz and agate, to mention a few of the most important ones. What is considered to be "precious" or "semi-precious" depends on the country, the time and the availability. Today there are only four really precious stones: the diamond, emerald, ruby and sapphire. Nearly all stones have found their way into purely ornamental jewelry, but, just as often, they have been sought after for their antidotal and occult powers.

The diamond is unrivalled as a precious stone. It was first mentioned in an old Indian tale over four thousand years ago and its first recorded use as an antidote was mentioned by the Roman scholar Pliny. The diamond, he wrote, can render *all* poisons harmless, and when dipped into wine or water will protect from "gout, jaundice and other maladies." When worn as an amulet it will protect from "plague and pestilence." Blood red agate and bloodstone, also observed nearly two thousand years ago, have lesser powers. Agate merely protects its owner against the bite of scorpion, and bloodstone, when powdered, can cure snakebite, stop bleeding and whiten blood-shot eyes. The amethyst has powers somehow connected with its color—that of the purple grape. If the figure of Bacchus, the god of wine, were inscribed on the stone and the stone then placed under the tongue its owner could ". . . consume a large vessel of wine without intoxication." If, instead of Bacchus, the "circle of the Sun were inscribed thereupon" it would protect its owner against the action of all poisons. Serpentine is speckled green like the skin of a serpent. When worn as an amulet it has the power to protect its owner against the bite of serpents, the sting of "noxious animals" and the effects of poison. Serpentine fashioned into a goblet will protect its owner by "bursting into a sweat" in the presence of a poison.

Even more remarkable is the power of some stones to detect and predict *changes* about to occur in the life of their owner.

The crimson ruby, for instance, is (ordinarily) good against witchcraft, pestilence and plague, but, when worn as an amulet the crimson will darken as illness approaches. The green emerald is (ordinarily) an antidote against poison. There's the story that an Arabian physician named Zoar instantly cured himself of the effects of a poisonous herb by placing one emerald on his stomach and one inside his mouth. Pliny adds that it will protect its owner against the venomous bites of serpents because sight of the emerald will "strike terror into the viper and cobra, such that their eyes leap out of their heads." But the emerald has the supernatural ability to warn its owner if any acts of treachery or deception are about to take place.

The topaz, normally a golden yellow, has the occult power to darken in the presence of poison, and the turquoise (also called the Turkish or Lucky Stone), when mounted in an amulet (an earring, ring, or pendant) has the power to completely change from its blue-green color should death approach the owner.

Stones of Animal Origin: the Bezoar,
Toadstone, Snakestone and Madstone

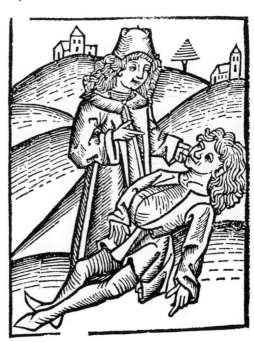

This drawing, first published in 1497, depicts the use of a bezoar stone as an antidote.

BEZOAR STONES

Bezoar stones originate as growths in the intestines of an animal. Calcareous materials accumulate around an irritant particle such as a fruit stone. In a sense it is like the pearl that forms layer upon layer around an irritant particle under the shell of a large mollusk. Bezoar stones come in various sizes and colors but most of them are yellowish and range in size between a hazelnut and an egg.

The bezoar stone was a favorite Eastern antidote for all poisons. It probably was first used in Arabia about 1100 A.D., but its fame spread so fast that it found its way to most ports of the world soon after. The name itself comes from its power as an antidote: bezoar literally means "the wind of the breeze of poison." That is, the bezoar simply "wafts away" the poison.

Bezoar stones come from cows, horses, certain species of ape and llamas, but the most prized of all bezoar stones (worth ten times its weight in gold during the Renaissance) came from the bowels of the Persian wild goat. It was sold in an 18th century English apothecary shop as an antidote to all poisons, under the name of "Lapis Bezoar Orientale."

The Dyaks, a tribe of head hunters now dwelling in the wilds of Central Borneo, routinely use a bezoar stone derived from the intestines of a wild boar. It resembles a round, whitish bird's egg and is so precious that the witchdoctor carries it carefully about in a soft skin pouch. On special occasions it is loaned to a distressed native, who is allowed to swallow it as part of the cure. (However, the native is restricted to quarters until the stone is recovered.) Bezoar stones in olden times were fashioned into jewelry, where they also served to keep the wealthy and influential safe from poison. Pope Innocent XI (who reigned between 1676 and 1689) was said to have an enormous collection of bezoar stone rings. Rings were a favorite mounting, but stones which dangled at the end of a chain were also in style in the Middle Ages. When on a chain the stone could be waved ceremoniously over water or wine before serving, in this way driving out the poison.

There were exceptions to belief in these remarkable powers, however. Ambroise Paré, physician to Charles IX, was one who took a jaundiced view of the bezoar stone. This was in spite of strong protest from the medical circles, which were filled with devoted believers. Paré tells of an instance when a Spanish nobleman came to the King to sell a bezoar stone, extolling its magic powers to work against the effects of all poisons. Paré was called to the Court, where he told the King that the whole story was poppycock, "as there were many kinds of poison and, hence, many antidotes needed to affect them." The King asked if there were any condemned prisoners in the dungeon, and as it turned out a palace cook was there, condemned to die for stealing two silver dishes from the palace galley. The cook was told that if he took a draught of poison and allowed the bezoar stone to be administered he would be pardoned. He was given the poison, and the stone . . . and in seven hours he was dead. The King promptly threw the bezoar stone into the fire. Paré's resistance to "progress" was in vain, for the sales remained at record highs both in numbers sold and prices charged.

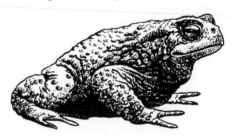

TOADSTONES

In the Middle Ages the toad was intimately associated with the monstrous basilisk, which could kill plants by a mere touch and smash rocks to smithereens with its hot breath. This was as wrong and unjust as believing there were Toad Demons covered with thick black fur, whose breath was deadly poison and whose body was so filled with venom that it was necessary for them to carry their own antidote to merely survive. Shakespeare in *As You Like It* alludes to the monstrous toad and its built-in antidote: "Sweet are the uses of adversity;/ Which, like the toad, ugly and venomous,/Wears yet a precious jewel in his head." A 16th century writer regarded the toad more kindly, for he wrote: "There is to be found in the heads of old and great toads a stone they called borax or stelon, which being used for a ring gives forwarning of venom."

A toadstone is any stone which resembles the shape or color of the toad and has the tradition of neutralizing poisons and curing the effects of bites or stings. The common variety is roundish and grey, tending toward blue. A more valuable kind is the elliptical stone, colored grey also but tending toward red, with deep reddish speckles. Most stones are mounted into rings in such a way that they touch the bare finger. In this manner they warn the owner that a poison is near by heating up against his finger. If the stone is used unmounted it can be placed directly over a bite, whereupon it will draw out all the poison. A particularly powerful stone is said to come from an uncommonly venomous toad. This stone can sweat and change color when it contacts a poison.

According to tradition, the chief claim to fame of the toadstone was that it was not "of the earth." It was obtained from the heads of old toads. Needless to say these stones are not taken from the head of a toad without substantial resistance. In his *Thousand Notable Things* the French writer Lupton describes a tricky procedure. The toads are first placed on a crimson cloth, "where they are much delighted, so that, while they stretch out themselves as it were in sport upon that cloth, they cast out the stone of their head, but instantly they sup it up again, unless it be taken from them through some secret hole in the same cloth." There is another less sporting method. The procedure calls for putting a well bruised and overgrown toad in an earthen pot, placing the pot in an ant-hill, covering it with earth, and allowing it to remain there until the ants have done their work and leave nothing but the bones—and the stones.

Bogus toadstones were a problem. It was necessary to tell a real one from a bogus one just as today a real diamond has to be distinguished from glittering glass. In the case of the toadstone, however, the expert was the toad itself. The stone was placed directly in front of the toad and both were closely observed. If the toad lunged violently toward the stone, as if to snatch it up, the stone was of high quality. The response of the toad indicated the antidotal power—if the toad was completely indifferent, this indicated a bogus stone.

Stones from other animals have powers almost as remarkable. The snakestone, obtained from the heads of Indian snakes, is dubbed *Cobra de Cabala*. When stuck over a venomous bite it draws out the poison, and when finished simply drops off. The source of the snakestone used by the American Indians is mineral, not animal. It is a stone which is only *shaped* like a snake and is supposed to possess lesser powers than the Cobra de Cabala.

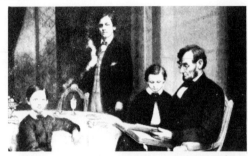

Even President Lincoln relied on the madstone's power as a cure for snakebite.

An Early American favorite was the madstone. There's little doubt that one of the most popular madstones was brought from Switzerland by an Italian cook and sold to a Kentucky farmer for a handsome American price. The stone itself measured a half inch (12 millimetres) across and an inch (25 millimetres) in length. It weighed two ounces (56 grams) and was bone white. In the 23 years that the farmer owned it he cured 59 cases of poisoning. It was placed over the bite where it soaked up poison until all the poison was out. Then it fell off. To restore the stone's powers, it was soaked in warm milk. The madstone was the Early American standard treatment for the bite of a mad dog (where it got its name) but it worked equally well for the bite of a snake. Abe Lincoln, in fact, took his son Robert to a madstone located in Terre Haute, Indiana after the lad was bitten by a snake.

The Land of Egypt

The world of ancient Egypt was an inseparable blend of mythology and real life. Amulets seemed to symbolize the union of mythology with everyday life. The Egyptians placed amulets everywhere. They were made of common stones, precious stones, wood, ivory, gold, silver, copper, bone, shell and wax. Most important though, they were inscribed with words of power from gods and magicians. It was through the inscription or word that power was transferred from the god to the wearer or owner of the amulet. The Arch-Demon Set, for example, was on a charm to ward off the bite of the scorpion.

The Egyptians believed that serpents, scorpions and other creatures were incarnations of evil spirits, which not only attacked the living but also the dead. Everyone was deathly

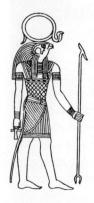

The Egyptians believed that even the gods were wary of venomous beasts—the sun god Ra (left) was nearly a snakebite victim, and Horus (right) died from a scorpion's sting.

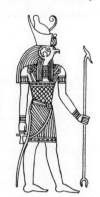

afraid of serpents, and to ward them off they placed amulets of stone containing a magic formula in each house and temple. Since the Egyptians believed strongly in the resurrection of the dead, they protected the corpses—preserving them as mummies and guarding them against deadly serpents with amulets in the tombs.

The gods (believed the Egyptians) were immune to the

attacks of serpents and other deadly animals because they possessed a certain virtue called the "fluid of life." But so evil were the serpents that even the sun god Ra nearly died of a bite—and Horus, the son of Isis, who was the wife and sister of the sun god Ra, actually did die by the bite of the scorpion. Fortunately Horus was brought back to life by a certain magic formula given to his mother, Isis, by the god of language and magic, Toth. It is these formulae—or parts of them—which were engraved on stone amulets and kept in Egyptian homes, tombs and temples. The stele called the Metternich Stele, one of the Cippi of Horus, the greatest amulets ever discovered, is an enormous polished black stone filled on front and back with magic formulae.

Fabulous Potions and Great Physicians

COLOPHON

One of the earliest physician-writers to recommend an antidote was Nicander of Colophon (2nd cent. B.C.). Besides being an outstanding botanist he was physician to Attalus, King of Pergamum and spark behind Colophon's accomplishments. The King gave Nicander anything he wanted, including a magnificent laboratory and an apparently unlimited supply of condemned criminals—all to be used for his experiments with poisons and antidotes. Colophon listed twenty-two poisonous plants, animals and minerals, including the noxious wolfsbane and hemlock and the deadly red toad. One of his favorite antidotes consisted of viper parts seasoned with aromatic roots and fruits such as ginger, cinnamon, myrrh, iris and gentian. His most workable antidote though consisted of warm oil and warm water with linseed tea. Invariably this caused his patient to throw up (probably its only secret of success).

PHILON OF TARSUS

Certainly one of the most celebrated and long-lived potions was the wild brew of the first century physician, Philon of Tarsus. His formula was inscribed on stone in symbolic Greek verse, a sort of code, but thanks to German and English translators we find that it was most likely a blend of several exotic or medicinal herbs, namely spikenard, henbane, pyrethrum, euphorbia and saffron (these are accompanied by mysterious instructions). In any event, the formula underwent changes but documents indicate that it surfaced again in 18th century London under the name of "Philonium Romanum." By this time the composition had changed to opium, pepper, ginger, caraway, honey, syrup and wine. Then a hundred years later, again in London, it came to be the "Confection of Opium." It may still be with us today, for in some parts of the world a mixture known as "Dover's Powder" is sold. A mixture of opium and ipecac (a common medicinal herb), it strongly resembles the "Confection," which was essentially opium.

PLINY THE ELDER

Pliny the Elder was not so much an experimenter as he was a scholar and writer. In the normal course of his work he discovered many "theriaca" (antidotes against serpents in particular and poisons in general). One which he believed to be among the first was "against the bites of all venomous animals" and was, like Philon's, inscribed on stone, this one located on the island of Cos, in the temple of Asklepios, the god of medicine. It contained "wild thyme, opoponax, aniseed, fennel, parsley, meum and ammi." These were to be beaten up with meal of fitches (*Ervum ervilla*), passed through a sieve, kneaded with wine, cut into lozenges of the weight of half a denarius (30 grams), one to be placed in three cyathi (5 ounces) of wine and swallowed. Another theriaca discovered by Pliny was that attributed to Zopyros, a Greek physician who lived around 80 B.C. The name given to Zopyros' great antidote was "Ambrosia," effective against the bite of all venomous animals except the cobra. It contained frankincense, golbanum, pepper and other aromatic substances with boiled honey. A piece the size of an Egyptian bean was to be taken, washed down with wine.

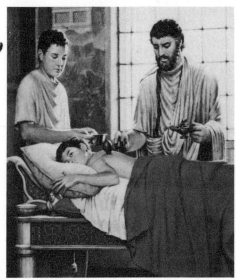

The ancient Greek physician Galen.

GALEN

Galen was undoubtedly one of the most famous of the ancient physicians. He was Greek, born in Pergamum in 129 A.D., studied and worked in Alexandria—the center of Greek medicine and science—and gained fame as the physician to the athletes and gladiators. As a writer he was most influential, for his book "The Method of Healing" was to become the basis for all medieval medicine. As an experimenter he compounded the "Nut Theriac," a remedy against bites and poisons. Taking it regularly, before meals, claimed Galen, would make the subject immune to the effects of all poisons. "It is composed of 4 figs, salt, nut and Ruta graveolens . . . of the leaves of Ruta 20 parts, the inner part of the nut

(2 nuts), salt 5 parts, dried fig 2 parts, all mixed into a kind of porridge."

This theriaca was to be taken with wine—unless, of course, the subject was someone for whom wine is forbidden. In this event, wrote Galen, a concoction of aniseed would do as well as wine. Galen also proposed a remedy for the bites of exceptionally venomous animals. To prepare this antidote: "Take the extract of the black henbane (sucran) and the white henbane (bang), 4 sikli each, castoreum, white pepper, costus, myrrh and opium, 1 siklus each, crush thin and suffuse with 3 ounces of sweet wine. Then warm in the sun until it solidifies. Of this pills are formed as big as an Egyptian pea (*Vicia faba*). Dosage—one pill to three ounces of sweet wine."*

MAIMONIDES

Maimonides was a prominent 12th century physician and personal physician to the Sultan of Egypt. At the request of the great Sultan, Maimonides devoted a great deal of time to antidotes and treatments for snakebite and food poisoning, with emphasis on snakebite. In both snakebite and food poisoning the victim had to first be prepared to receive the antidote. In food poisoning the first step was to cause the victim to vomit, to rid the body of as much poison as fast as possible. Following the stomach purge, soup with bread crumbs and much butter and cream was to be served, and this kept in the stomach for just one hour. *Then* the antidote was to be administered. Before administering the antidote to a snakebite victim a more complicated routine was necessary. First the region above the wound was to be tied off as fast as possible to prevent spreading of the poison. Then another person was to cut directly above the wound and suck out the poison—taking care to coat his mouth with olive oil first.

*Sussman, Muntner (ed.), *The Medical Writings of Moses Maimonides*, © 1966, J. B. Lippincott Co.

Suction cups could be substituted (but they were seldom available). Following this procedure the victim was to vomit and empty his stomach. *Then* the antidote was to be administered. After this a medicine was to be applied to the wound and allowed to draw the poison out of the body. If the victim responded well the treatment was a success. If not, he was beyond the powers of Maimonides' first aid and the victim was referred to a specialist.

Maimonides compiled a list of remedies for drawing out poisons. For a simple remedy one of the following ingredients could be chosen: ocimum basilicum, sulphur, duck excrement, goat dung, salt or any type of onion. The chosen ingredient was to be crushed and kneaded with honey, then made into a plaster and applied to the clean wound. This remedy would draw poisons directly out of the wound.

Maimonides selected various compounded medicines from the writings of ancient and medieval physicians. A favorite of Maimonides was the great 10th century Arabian physician named Rhazes, who told all in his *Secret of Secrets*. At this period in Islamic history there was the belief that all questions in biology and medicine had been answered and there was nothing left to be solved. The remedy suggested by Rhazes during this period of final enlightenment was to be effective against all poisonous bites. He stated the composition: "dried shelled nut, grossly ground salt, one part, dried leaves of Ruta graveolens, one sixth each, white figs in a quantity equal to all the rest. This is divided into portions somewhat bigger than a nut and one portion taken at a time."

Avicenna (980–1077 A.D.) followed Rhazes and became the most famous scientist of the Islamic world. He wrote about everything, but noteworthy among his accomplishments was his "electuary," effective against all bites. It was prepared with seven different herbs kneaded in skimmed honey.

Maimonides recorded simple and powerful remedies effective against all deadly poisons entering the body, "whether by mouth or by bite." They were the bezoar, the emerald and the citrus seed. The bezoar had to be of animal origin; the emerald "juicily green," translucent, reduced to a fine powder, and 9 grains were to be taken in wine or water; and the citrus seed was to be prepared by peeling off the outer layer, crushing it and consuming up to 2 drams in wine or water.

GRIFFIN CLAW AND UNICORN HORN

Certain amulets, usually fashionable goblets, had the power to detect poisons or send off a warning alarm.

The unicorn of mythology had the head of a horse, the feet of an elephant and the tail of a boar—and a single spiralling black horn coming straight out of its head. The unicorn horn was the antidote to all poisons in food or wine. As Aristotle claimed, anyone who drank from a goblet of unicorn horn was protected against all poisons. He could drink from the vessel either before or after the poisoning and still be immune to its effects. Queen Elizabeth I, James I and Charles I each had a unicorn horn in their possession. (Elizabeth's was worth over a hundred thousand English pounds.) Those of lesser rank owned mere fragments of unicorn horn, which they simply dipped into wine and water as a routine precaution. The obvious question arises: If the unicorn was mythical, what was it that these affluent Europeans were using? Probably ivory from the horns or tusks of the rhinoceros, elephant or narwhal. (The narwhal is a pale-skinned type of whale that grows to a length of 15 feet (4.5 metres) and, in the male, has a 9-foot (3-metre) horn or "tooth" protruding from its head.) The Norsemen were said to have sold these tusks or horns to Europeans as "genuine horn of unicorn."

The Chinese fashioned highly ornamental goblets from the horn of the Indian rhinoceros. The palaces of the great Eastern Emperors were never without the services of these cups, as poisons were frequently used by assassins. The horn of the

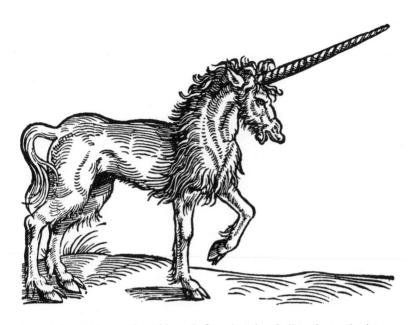

The rich and the royal paid heavily for what they believed was the horn of the unicorn (above, as pictured in 1551); what they were getting was probably the horn of the narwhal (below, as pictured in 1578).

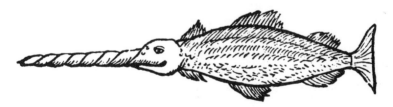

rhinoceros was not an antidote so much as a poison alarm. If a poisonous liquid was poured into the cup and allowed to stand for a short time, the cup would sweat and the outside would change color.

During the Middle Ages antelope horns, also called "Griffin Claws," were fashioned into goblets. (The Griffin was the half-eagle, half-lion which drew the mythical chariots of the gods Zeus, Apollo and Nemesis across the skies. The Griffin also

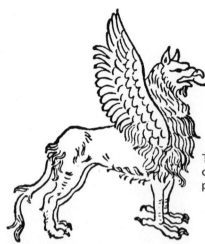

The claws of the griffin were coveted as indicators of poisonous potions.

guarded the gates to the Garden of Eden.) Goblets of Griffin Claws had the rare ability to change color when a poison drew near.

Horn of Cerastes is the rarest material of all. It comes from two small horn-like projections above the eyes of a certain type of snake. A knife handle made of the Horn of Cerastes is said to froth if it touches poisoned food or drink.

Electrum, an alloy of gold and silver, is more spectacular than the ivory-like materials comprising most of the palace goblets. When a poison is within the goblet of electrum, circular rainbows begin to dance on the liquid's surface while the liquid itself sparkles and hisses as if it were on fire.

The horns on the head of the cerastes snake were made into knife handles.

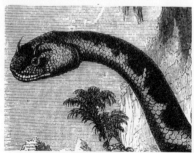

MITHRIDATICUM

Potions as antidotes have also been popular through the ages. To King Mithridates VI Eupator we owe at least a very different approach to the problem of poisoning. Mithridates, King of Pontus in Asia Minor during the first century B.C., was deathly afraid of being poisoned. As a precaution against attempts on his life he tried to make himself into a walking universal antidote by taking a little of each kind of poison every day, thereby building up an immunity. To cover the whole gamut of poisons he sent his men all over the world gathering poisons to be tried out by him—but only after they were sampled by slaves. He also tried to develop a universal antidote that could be taken like any ordinary dose of medicine. His formula (discovered after his death) was called "Mithridaticum," and was said to contain half a hundred ingredients and consist mostly of viper flesh.

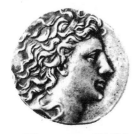

King Mithridates VI Eupator of Pontus (132–63 B.C.).

The story of Mithridates' end is most unusual for a man of his particular ambitions. The King was a political fanatic who violently opposed the Roman takeover in the Near East. To gain his objectives and get at the Romans he overthrew his mother in 110 B.C., seized the reins of government and proceeded to massacre over 80,000 Italian settlers in and around Asia Minor. To Rome this was a treacherous act of war and armies were sent out after Mithridates. When after many years they finally succeeded in subduing him the defeated ruler committed suicide by taking an enormous overdose of poison!

The universal antidote called Mithridaticum somehow survived the centuries and arose again in the guise of the Theriaca of Venice (also called the Treacle), a mysterious mixture containing some 61 ingredients. The Bologna (Italian) version of the theriaca was compounded in a sacred place under the watchful eyes of city officials and university professors. The purpose, of course, was to ensure a potent mixture, useful against the Great Plague then raging through Europe and surrounding countries. (The Plague had to be respected: it was known to wipe out half a city in one season.)

It's likely that the Treacle was not very different from the famous concoction of the 16th century physician, Pietro Andrea Malthiolus, or that of Mithridates. Malthiolus' preparation had 251 ingredients (probably the most complex theriaca in history). Among the ingredients were dried viper, pearls, red coral and emeralds. This mixture, like the Treacle of Venice, required ceremonious attention in the courtyard of a monastery.

OLD LONDON "QUACKS"

The Quacks of Old London were the most eloquent sorcerers (and sorceresses) in all of history. They addressed audiences with polish and style:

"Gentlemen and Ladies,

"Behold this little vial, which contains in its narrow bounds what the whole universe cannot purchase, if sold to its true value . . . drawn from the *hearts* of *Mandrakes, Phoenix livers, Tongues* of *Mermaids* and distilled by contracted *Sunbeams* . . . Gentlemen, If any of you present was at Death's door, here's this, my Divine Elixir, will give you Life again.

'This will recover whole fields of Slain,

And all the Dead shall rise and fight again.' "

(And so on and on.)

The *Famous Pills* of one Richard Matthews, a well known London quack, were claimed to be an antidote to all poisons.

Matthews claimed there was "a gentleman who drank 200 grains of opium at one draught, then swallowed a pill and yet is in good health." Matthews died in 1662 but in 1663 his wife issued a treatise called "True Receipt for the *Famous Pills* made by Richard Matthews." The composition as revealed by Mrs. Matthews was as follows: "Tartar, salt peter, heated together in an iron kettle, stirred well and allowed to cool. This salt is then mixed with Oyl of Turpentine and stirred, and allowed to stand for six months, then opium and hellebire [hellebore] is added, the whole being well beaten into a paste with a little more turpentine."

"NEGRO CAESAR'S CURE FOR POISON"

Universal antidotes in Early America lacked all of the European pomp and ceremony. In 1750 the General Assembly of Carolina allowed the publication of "Negro Caesar's Cure for Poison." Caesar gained his freedom in exchange for his formula—which was made from the roots of plantain and wild horehound, boiled in water, and taken three mornings "while the patient is fasting." As a safeguard the clever Caesar pointed out that if the remedy didn't work it was a sign "that the patient had either not been poisoned," or, if he died, that the poisoning had been accomplished "by such poison as Caesar's antidote will not remedy."

A DUEL OF POISONS

Strange though it may seem neither poisons nor their antidotes need be material. They can be psychological . . . or psychic! In *Treasury of Secretes* the ancient Persian poet Nizami dramatizes the power of pure suggestion. His poem describes a poison-antidote duel between two court physicians. The two physicians developed such an intense rivalry that they chose to settle matters by a duel—an ordeal by poison. The physicians agreed that each should take a poison given him by his opponent and that this poison should be countered by an antidote of the victim's choice. Physician number one prepared a draught "the fierceness of which would have melted stone." Physician number two downed the goblet-full and took his antidote—nulling the poison in an instant. It was now the turn of the first physician to accept the challenge. The second physician walked to the garden, picked a rose, breathed an incantation over it, and challenged his opponent to smell it. At that very instant the opponent fell down dead. In Nizami's poem:

"Through this rose which the spell breather had given him
Fear over mastered the foe and he gave up the ghost,
That one by treatment expelled the poison from his body,
While this one died of a rose from fear."

Rise of the Celebrated Poison Cults

Primitive man and his poisons exist in a timeless world. It is next to impossible to affix specific dates and times to events in the societies of the Bushmen or the Malayans. The situation is somewhat different in the cradles of civilization such as Babylonia and Egypt, and the great civilizations of later times.

THE PENALTY OF THE PEACH

Mysteries of ancient Egyptian medicines and poisons came to us through eight medical papyri, all written somewhere between 1900–1100 B.C. The longest is known as the Ebers Papyrus, a scroll some 20 yards (18 metres) long, which lists the well known drugs and poisons of that era. One of the eight scrolls contains what Egyptologists believe to be the first written record of a lethal preparation. Translated, the famous sentence reads: "Pronounce not the name of I.A.D. under penalty of the peach." This is taken to refer to the then new technique called distillation, and the process refers to distilling cyanide from the crushed seeds of a peach.

Better known are the later periods in Greece, Persia and the Far East.

In Greece around 500 B.C. we find an amazing variety of poisons: arsenic, antimony, mercury, gold, silver, copper, hemlock, aconite, colchicum and henbane. In Persia of the same era we find a similar arsenal of poisons, and, if we are to believe some of the stories, the Persians knew how to use them for sinister purposes.

There's the story that Queen Parysatis, who reigned beside Artaxerxes II (405–359 B.C.), poisoned her daughter-in-law Satira with the poisoned-knife trick. She coated one side of the blade with venom before serving "a bird" between herself and Satira. The Queen was careful to eat the part off the clean side of the knife. She survived the dinner. Satira didn't.

In earlier periods before our era the Hindus were as fanatic and secretive as were the Egyptians. Hindus listed the well known poisons: aconite, arsenic, lead, opium, and many plant poisons. One not so common was a mysterious fungus, *Mucor phycomyces*. Mixed with water this fungus could attach itself to the throat and grow slowly. In two weeks the poisons given off by the fungus choked the victim, as if by strangulation.

A POISONER'S PARADISE

During our own A.D. era the popularity of poisons ebbed for a time but reached unprecedented heights during the Renaissance, the 14th to the 17th century. Poisons became popular because poisoning someone was very easy: just sprinkle a little poison powder on food, water or wine . . . and wait. Seldom would questions be asked. In palaces and the households of the wealthy there were food tasters and magic amulets, but still there was no limit to some people's imagination. It is said that a 15th century court physician murdered the King of Naples by putting poison on the lips of his daughter (also the King's mistress). When she kissed the King it was for his last time. In England a favorite trick was to dust powder into the victim's gloves. This method took a little longer but it did work. Itching powder was sometimes substituted for the arsenic usually dusted into gloves—victims have been known to scratch themselves to death.

In 1700 the new scientific revolution introduced the science of poisons called toxicology. This was to be the science that ended the rule of the poisoner. Convictions were expected to increase, yet 100 years later, in 1800, there was no noticeable change in the status of the poisoner. Poisoners went about their trade—and the art of poisoning, as usual, was still a great mystery to the spectator public. There seemed to be no defense against the wily poisoner. With convictions based on the chemical analysis of poisons still nonexistent in 1800 it is easy to see why the early and late Renaissance, several hundred years *before* this time, were a poisoner's paradise.

Cult of the Professional Poisoner

Italy of the Renaissance was a mecca for poisoners of all rank. The school of Venice was one of the poisoners' schools set into operation before the 16th century. We can only guess what happened to its "graduates" but it is known that the poisoning madness of Italy in these years reached such proportions that it even became a formal method for the assassination of officials. There appeared in the government of Venice a Secret Circle. Anyone who displeased the Circle in any way—whether Emperor, Prince or Pope—was simply removed. There are official records which give the gruesome details of what went on behind the closed doors of the "Council of Ten," the "Circle." This sinister group met to discuss who should be removed and (possibly) why. Then they took a vote for or against and sealed the contract as they would any business deal. After the contract was carried out the official

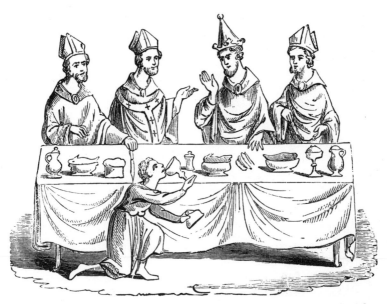

Wine tasters had a dangerous job in the 15th century—they tested for the presence of poison, not the quality of the beverage.

records were completed by the single word "Factum" opposite the new victim's name. Professional poisoners were used to carry out most of these contracts for the Council. They bid like any modern businessman might.

A typical bidder was a Franciscan brother, John of Ragusa. On December 15, 1548 he described his services to the Council; that is, he presented his selection of poisons and methods, and the prices. The fees, of course, depended mostly on the rank of the victim. For example: "For the King of Spain 150 ducats [a ducat is now very roughly $5 or £3]—including travel expenses; for the Duke of Milan, 60 ducats; for the Pope, 100 ducats, . . ." Even more, he boasted that he would remove anyone the council could name.

DEADLY SCHOOLING

The Roman school was no less prominent than the one in Venice. (The word school isn't meant to imply classrooms and the rest. It refers to knowledge circulated about in a small group of people, usually quite unofficially.) Knowledge was more widespread and all that was needed was

- the need: perhaps to resolve some personal problem involving an enemy.
- the poison: usually belladonna, aconite, hellebore or arsenic—obtainable in much the same way liquor was during the American Prohibition.
- the method: for unsophisticated poisoners this could amount to simply "sprinkling it on" but for those of more sophisticated bent there were personal instructors and books.

"Poison Formulas" by Baptista Parta was published in 1589. His most powerful formula was a mixture of "aconite, taxus bacceta, caustic lime, arsenic, bitter almonds and powdered glass"—blended with honey and rolled into a pill as big as a hazelnut. How to use it was apparently up to the reader. In another formula he specified a poison especially for sleeping persons. For this mix "hemlock juice, bruised stramonium, belladonna and opium." Place the blend in a box with a perfectly fitting lid and allow it to ferment for three days, he ordered, then uncover it and place it directly under the intended victim's nose.

THE BORGIA ATROCITIES

Historians believe that the Borgia family was associated with some of the most morbid crimes of the later Renaissance. Originally the Borgias came from Spain ("Borgia" is the Latin version of the Spanish "Borja"). When Nicholas V, known as the humanist Pope, died in 1455 A.D., the Borgias were started on their way to papal history. Calixtus III (formerly Alonso

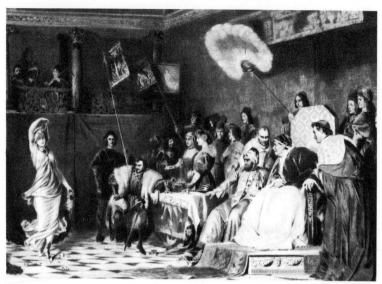

The infamous Lucretia Borgia dances for Pope Pius III and her brother Cesare.

de Borja) succeeded Nicholas V to become Pope. His generosity (to his own family) was exceeded by none. He showered them with appointments and estates. One appointment was that of Rodrigo Borgia, then 26, as Cardinal in the Church. Then on August 6, 1458 Calixtus III died and Pius II succeeded him. Rodrigo flourished under the overly permissive Pius II. Once, for example, Rodrigo held an orgy. He was reprimanded by Pope Pius II: "Dear Son: . . . we have learned that the most licentious dances were performed, that no amorous allurement was wanting, and that you behaved like a man unmindful of his estate . . ." With little to be feared, Rodrigo's conduct continued and soon all Rome knew of Cardinal Rodrigo Borgia's "liaison" with a young woman called Vanozza de' Cattanel . . . and their 4 children born between 1474 and 1482: Cesare, Juan, Joffre and Lucretia. When Rodrigo became Pope Alexander VI he expressed high hopes for his 4 children—

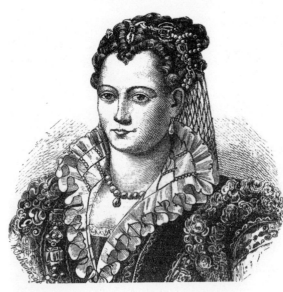

Lucretia Borgia
(1480–1519).

especially Cesare, who he thought should mark himself for a life in the Church. Unfortunately, Alexander VI had no control over his children whatever. Stories circulated about Cesare in particular. Once, in a fit of jealousy over an attendant in his sister's household, he attacked and pursued the attendant with a dagger—all the way to the Pontifical Chamber, where he stabbed the poor fellow to death, blood spattering onto the Pontifical robe. But Cesare did become Cardinal of Valentia in Spain before he was 18.

There is the story that the Pope commanded Cesare to escort the King of France while the King was a guest of Italy. No one knows whether the French King was always so security conscious or whether Cesare's reputation preceded him, but a historian of the era wrote this about the King's visit: "The King sat on his bed, had his boots removed and put on his pattons; he went out of the chamber where the table had been placed, settled near the fire, had his beard combed, and then began to sup . . . The King drank from a golden cup, and wine was poured into the cup, one of his men, who had a gold chain, took from it a piece of horn, which is an antidote, and turned it about these cups, then gave some wine to the wine-taster, and some of this wine was put in another cup; and four physicians had to judge if the wine was good for his Majesty the King. And the same was done with the dishes . . ."

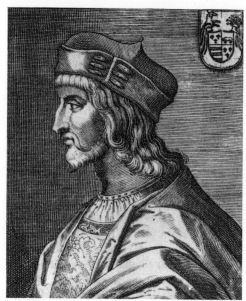

Cesare Borgia
(c.1475–1507).

CESARE'S "LA CANTARELLA"

Rumors had Cesare carrying out poisonings for the Pope: two in particular, a member of the Turkish royalty named Prince Djem and the Duke of Grandier. Poisoning was a routine crime in Italy of the Renaissance. When passing a church on the way to a crime, criminals stopped to make the sign of the cross and asked the Madonna for her blessing in their upcoming venture.

But Cesare Borgia was no ordinary criminal. He had position and wealth. This included a special room to prepare his concoctions (only he, the Pope and Lucretia were ever allowed to enter it) and advice from unusual persons. One such was a Spanish monk who gave him his precious formula, known as "La Cantarella" (only the Monk, it is said, knew the antidote). Cesare spoke of an incantation he used to put the finishing touches on his evil brew. It went: "God said 'Let there be light': And there was light. We Borgias say: 'Let there be night': And night it shall be." No one knows what his formula really was. Records are confusing, but according to one Carelli, who was physician to Charles VI and quite a reputable person, the following is a description of Cesare's "La Cantarella": "The abdominal viscera of a sow which was poisoned by arsenic are covered over by arsenic powder and putrefaction is allowed to proceed until liquids flow from it. These are concentrated by evaporation until they constitute a white powder—which is called 'La Cantarella'."

"AQUA TOFFANA"

The woman called Toffana operated the Naples Route. When brought to justice in 1709 she admitted murdering 600 people (including 2 Popes). One of her secrets was that she rubbed arsenic into the joints of freshly slaughtered swine, then put the juice into her confections. Her method of doing business was almost charming—and legal (if anyone cared). She put her solutions into fancy little vials and sold them under the names of Saints and other labels, such as "Aqua Toffana." The vials were for women who wanted to improve their complexions, as strong solutions of arsenic were known to do. Except the woman could choose to use the solution as a "spouse remover" as well. As little as 5 drops in a drink of wine or water . . . and a new husband was on the way.

THE MARCHIONESS DE BRINVILLIERS

About the time Madame Toffana was poisoning in Italy one of history's most charming poisoners, Madame de Brinvilliers, was doing much the same in France. The Marchioness was little, graceful, blue-eyed and modest . . . and of noble origins. Nobility seemed to give her a license for her madness. She had a consuming interest in poisons and preferred exact experiments. The best training involved human beings, of course, and these were readily available at a nearby hospital, where she "ministered to the poor sick." Her patients, however, tended to die rather soon after she offered her services (the hospital didn't mind: they needed the room). The Madame had the best of sources for all the poison she needed: an apothecary operated by the King's own pharmacist, which she visited in a black cloth disguise to keep her activities secret.

Over the years she used poisons on servants and members of the family with the same coldness that she "ministered to the poor sick." Even after her father was in the Bastille, the most infamous prison in France's history, she continued to poison him—slowly and systematically, watching when she could every agonizing move he made, with never so much as a twinge of pity. The only comment she had was that she thought he "would never get to the end of it." Her list of victims included two brothers, various attempts on the life of her sister-in-law and even her own daughter (because she was "so stupid").

The wheels of justice finally caught up with her and convicted her of all her vicious crimes (she confessed all). The evidence that convicted her included letters and descriptions of poisonings, accidentally found in a small casket owned by a former husband. The husband had died in poverty and it was a regulation of the State that all property belonging to a debtor be impounded.

On the final day of her life, as she sat on the scaffold looking at a courtyard dotted with the heads of "all those vulgar people" waiting to see her beheaded on the guillotine, her face convulsed and it was this horrible grimace that was captured by the painter Le Brun. The famous sketch he made still hangs in the Louvre in Paris.

Poisoning in More Recent Times

Poisoners like Madame de Brinvilliers went confidently on for many years. There was an endless parade of "spouse removers," "inheritance powders" and personalized concoctions. True, some cases came to court but this was more accidental than ordinary. Those that came to court involved outright bungling, an unbelievable weight of circumstantial evidence, or plain confessions by accomplices. For the most part poisoners had their ancient free run until 1813. That's when forensic chemistry was born.

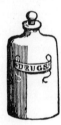 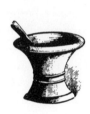 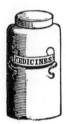

DOCTORS OF POISON

Ten years later, in 1823, the first poisoner was convicted on the basis of a direct chemical analysis of the internal organs of the victim. It happened that this poisoner was a doctor, the first of many medical men to be convicted poisoners. Morphine, opium, and strychnine were most frequently used by doctors. Two of the most famous cases involved the clever use of newer poisons. The first was a French doctor named Count de la Pommerais. He was convicted by a chemical analysis revealing the poison digitalis. The second was that of an English doctor named George Lamson. In 1882 Doctor Lamson was convicted of using aconite to murder his crippled nineteen-year-old brother-in-law for his inheritance. There's the story that Lamson was a student of the famous toxicologist Sir Robert Christison. In a lecture one day Sir Christison stated that aconite was an undetectable poison. As a good student would, Lamson put this into his notes. Unfortunately for Lamson, between the time of his note taking and the actual murder aconite *did* become detectable by chemical methods.

Doctors were unusually well qualified as poisoners, but poisoning belonged to the greater public too. Renaissance sophistication had disappeared but, chemical analysis or not, convictions were still hit and miss. Most poisonings involved the ever popular arsenic, often administered with uncommon crudity. Following arsenic were: laudanum given in coffee (laudanum is a mixture of opium and alcohol), chloroform, tartar emetic (antimony), and cantharides. The last named poison, sometimes called "Spanish Fly," is usually not intended for murder but is so extraordinarily potent that an overdose is easily taken by the victim or given by someone attempting to arouse a member of the opposite sex to passion.

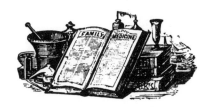

Poisons and Modern Biology

> Scientists at the forefront of modern toxicology continue to refine new techniques for detecting infinitesimal amounts of poison (a useful skill for criminologists) and evaluating the toxicity of newly discovered compounds. A scientific explanation of "How can so little poison be so deadly?" follows, along with the most effective "universal antidote" found to date in the laboratory.

Trends in Poison Science

Sputnik and the other Russian space miracles touched off a war of challenge in the field of instruments. New developments in the fields of microelectronics and computers have improved such instruments as the microscope and spectrograph immeasurably. Detections as low as "ppt" (parts per trillion) are common in analytical instruments today. Even a single atom has been photographed—not in the ordinary sense (an atom is too small to reflect light waves) but as a "representation," a pattern caused by the lone atom itself.

> While scientific instruments used throughout the world are equally sensitive the units of measure are not the same throughout. The system of numeration used in the United States (used in this book) calls the number 1,000,000,000 a *billion* while the British system calls this a *milliard*. Similarly, the number 1,000,000,000,000 is an American *trillion*, but it is only called a *billion* in the British system.

Modern research efforts are being directed toward different aspects of the whole problem of poisons. There is some work now to predict whether new substances will or will not be poisonous to humans—even *before* they are made or discovered. Toxicity studies in the past were not always up to the task.

Some, for example, showed a substance to be harmless. Alone, and at the higher concentration levels, the particular substance was often harmless as claimed, but in combination with other chemicals it might not be. Some present programs of research study the poisonous effects of cadmium, bismuth, mercury and other elements and their compounds in such a detailed manner that changes produced by poisons in different portions of a single cell can be determined. Microscopes now routinely study the inner parts of single cells. Analysis of material involved in crimes or of samples taken from victims is so refined that almost any poison can be detected at a very low level of concentration.

The New Criminalistics

It's well known that if a criminologist knows what he's looking for he will find it, if it's there. The new instruments and improved techniques ensure its detection. The problem is that although routine screening tests are performed there are just too many possible poisons to test for more than a few of these possibilities. In the 1940's there were 60 possible poisons that could be used by poisoners. Most of these were preparations based on poisonous plants. In the 1950's, along with the instrument explosion came the chemistry explosion. Pharmaceutical houses discovered ways of slightly rearranging the constituents of the complex molecules with which they were dealing. The shift of an atom or a small group of atoms from one place to another, taking one away here, adding two there— all these little tricks changed the properties of a substance just a little. The basic poison possibilities, now about 5000, could in this way be extended to perhaps 250,000. Needless to say, painstaking search by criminologists for unknown members of such a group is impossible. Almost any poison *could* be found in the body if we only knew which one to look for, but the new instruments are wonder machines only for problems which are "spelled out." Luckily the practical possibilities for the poisoner haven't changed much. The number of available poisons is still about the same because the newest drugs or "experimental" poisons are not easily available. Nor has the situation changed much for the detective. He still starts with a suspicion and follows his hunches.

To look for poisons a sample is taken from the victim: fluid contents if the victim is living or samples from various parts of the body if not. Each organ or tissue is packaged in a separate, absolutely clean, plastic container. No additives are used for proper preservation—only refrigeration. Knowing which organ the poison was in helps narrow down the search. Samples include virtually everything thought to have a bearing on the case, which may include chips of glass or metal or paint, bits of blood and fragments of hair.

NEUTRON ACTIVATION

One of the most sensitive of all the modern methods of analysis is *neutron activation*. The sample to be analyzed is placed in an experimental nuclear reactor or a cyclotron and bombarded by a massive beam of neutrons. Say the sample is a pinch of powder with the elements indium and manganese present at minute levels, or several strands of hair containing arsenic. The indium, manganese, and arsenic will be changed to radioactive forms called *isotopes*. Arsenic isotope will give off radiation by which it and it alone can be picked up by the analyzing instruments. Manganese and indium are detected at their own characteristic settings. The method of neutron activation is so extraordinarily sensitive that detections at the parts per trillion level have been made. Using this technique a few strands of Napoleon's hair were analyzed. They were taken from a locket containing a few snips taken shortly before death. Analysis showed an arsenic level of 13 parts per million, fifteen times higher than it should have been. The conclusion was thereby reached that Napoleon was poisoned by arsenic

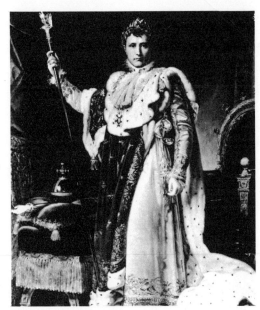

Did Napoleon die of natural causes? Modern science says no—he was poisoned.

served in his meals during the latter days or weeks of his exile. The method is sensitive enough to analyze segments of a single hair, starting at the root. In this way the degree of poisoning can be correlated with time. The older method, by way of contrast, would not only be time consuming but would have required dissolving a thousand hairs for a one-time-only try.

RADIO IMMUNE TECHNIQUE

The radio immune technique, a relative newcomer now used in forensic laboratories, is important because of the modern concern with drug abuse and overdose. The purpose is to measure the concentration of drugs in tissues. A radioactive solution is added to a specimen which is known to contain a particular drug. This causes a chemical reaction and, by measuring the level of radioactivity remaining after the reaction is complete, scientists can determine the amount of the drug present in the original specimen.

A Little Goes a Long Way

As little as two tenths of one milligram of saxitoxin will kill a 200 pound (90 kilogram) man. This is the weight of 1/100th of a drop of water, barely visible to the naked eye. How can two tenths of one milligram kill an adult man? One who weighs 500 million times as much as the dose of poison?

Monkey Wrenches in the Biological Machinery

Put another way the previous question might become: "If a man were an enormous machine how big a monkey wrench would it take to jam up the works?"

TURNED-OFF ENZYMES

An enzyme is really a substance that changes one compound into another—by its mere presence. Speaking very generally an enzyme is any substance which in very minute amounts exerts a great effect on a living system. Enzymes are essential to important functions of the living cell. The enzyme called maltase, for example, has one important task in the cell: to take water and other materials and use them to make the simple sugar called glucose.

ARCHITECTURAL PECULIARITIES

An enzyme is a kind of protein and, like all proteins, it is made up of a complicated arrangement of atoms of the elements carbon, hydrogen, nitrogen, oxygen, sulphur and other metals at trace levels. A typical protein is the substance found in all red blood cells—hemoglobin. Its formula is $C_{3032} H_{4816} O_{872} N_{780} S_8 Fe_4$. This means that 3032 atoms of carbon are strung into a long curled-up chain and that 4816 atoms of hydrogen, 872 of oxygen, 780 of nitrogen, 8 of sulphur and 4 of iron form various short branches, shooting off the carbon chain at various points along its length. There's one very important architectural fact about most proteins that are also enzymes. They are "globular" rather than "linear." This means they have loops and twists and are delicate for this reason. Each loop and twist has a meaning and a purpose. It is also a fact that loops and twists are easily destroyed by the protein's two greatest enemies: heat and poison.

KEY ENZYMES

Each enzyme usually has only one job to do, so there must be roughly as many different chemical reactions going on as there are enzymes. The liver cell, for example, is supposed to house about 50,000 different enzymes and carry on as many chemical reactions. It is by far the most complex cell in the human body.

Some enzymes come in relatively large quantities and others are present in minuscule amounts, while some enzymes have apprentice rank jobs and others are like key personnel. When the enzyme cytochrome is destroyed by cyanide, for instance, the cells can no longer *use* oxygen even though it is there in great abundance. Cytochrome is a "key" enzyme in this scheme of comparison.

In brief: *Monkey wrench number one* in the body machinery is the turned-off enzyme. The process of damping down or turning off enzyme activity—known more technically as "enzyme inhibition"—can cause disability and death. If a poison directs itself to an enzyme which is *both* a key enzyme and is present in minuscule amounts, the body machinery is in deep trouble.

NUMBERS MAKE THE DIFFERENCE

Poisons can wipe out a vital enzyme only if there are enough of the poison molecules present—comparable to having a dozen rioters for every policeman.

Cyanide

A fatal dose of cyanide involves about 50 milligrams, approximately the weight of a postage stamp. Yet this dosage contains close to 10 billion, billion molecules. The number of cells in the human body number about a hundred trillion (or a hundred thousand billion) cells. This puts the number of cyanide molecules at about ten to one, compared to the total number of body cells. Cyanide kills by turning off an enzyme the cell needs to use oxygen from the blood. This particular enzyme, cytochrome, is vital to the very last stage in the process for using oxygen. A victim of cyanide poisoning has blood so loaded with oxygen that his face is pink. Oxygen appears at the cell door (so to speak) but the cyanide won't let it in.

Carbon Monoxide

Carbon monoxide works somewhat differently than cyanide. In this instance it is not a vital enzyme that is turned off but rather a whole-body function that is damped down. Again numbers help answer the question "Why does it take so little of a poison to kill a man?"

Carbon monoxide is a common gas that comes from car exhausts, defective camp stoves, and a thousand and one other places where burning is not complete. It is always in the air and hovers above freeways at several parts per million—a dangerous level if we're required to breath it for hours at a time.

It's dangerous because it's attracted to the hemoglobin of our own blood three hundred times as strongly as oxygen. This means that in a contest it will almost always win its place on the hemoglobin molecule. Normally the hemoglobin of the red blood cells picks up oxygen as it passes through the lungs and moves it through the tiny capillaries to the oxygen-starved cells of the body. Oxygen attaches loosely to hemoglobin and so is easily "dropped off" where needed. Not so when carbon monoxide combines with the hemoglobin. It forms a tightly bound combination and oxygen can no longer be dropped off where it is needed. Cells therefore die and if there are enough of the carbon monoxide molecules the body suffers death by suffocation—just as surely as if the victim were strangled.

Breathing a few parts per million of carbon monoxide in the

air above a freeway can be overcome by the body, in time. A fatal dose would involve breathing an atmosphere containing 1/10 of one per cent carbon monoxide, and this for close to three hours. In three hours half the red blood cells would be bound up and immobilized and not enough oxygen would reach the body cells to maintain life. In these three hours of (normal) breathing the victim breathes in about 10,000 billion, billion molecules of carbon monoxide. For a normal man having about 25 billion red blood cells all told, this is a ratio of 400 billion molecules of carbon monoxide for every red cell in the body. The "rioters" outnumber the "policemen" by quite a margin.

In brief: *Monkey wrench number two* in the biological machinery is the overwhelming number of molecules in even the tiniest speck of matter. And the fact that a few molecules can do so much damage—by either cancelling out vital enzymes (as they do to the cytochrome in cyanide poisoning) or by eliminating vital body functions (such as the oxygen transport system in carbon monoxide poisoning).

SIGNAL WIRES AND FAULTY SWITCHES

The nervous system of a human being works something like the electrical system of a complex machine. Signals are sent through the biological "wiring" of interconnected nerves in order to control the movement of the muscles which are distant from the control function in the brain. If these signals fail to get to the muscles, or if the message is distorted, then the body cannot function efficiently and, in extreme cases, death is the result.

Carrying a message from the brain to the hand, for instance, is not quite as straightforward as conducting electricity through a metal wire. In the body the impulse must be transferred from one nerve to another, and then from the nerve to the muscle. The connections are not direct—there is a gap between the nerves, or the nerve and the muscle, and the complex reactions which occur in this gap are particularly vulnerable to disruption by poison.

If we had a powerful microscope we could see the details of the nerve/muscle junction, looking like the illustration shown here. The gap shown in the drawing is a battleground between two warring fluids. One of these allows the nerve impulse to pass along, the other works to stop the impulse by destroying the first fluid.

Tiny vesicles of acetylcholine (one of the two warring fluids) are made and stored in the nerve ending. The nerve impulse causes several of the vesicles to rupture and flow into the gap. When the acetylcholine attaches itself to the membrane on the opposite side of the gap it changes the membrane's condition and sends an impulse into the muscle. (This is success: it is doing what it was meant to do.)

If the acetylcholine now stayed in the gap there would be a continual stimulation of the muscle, something like short-circuit conditions in the electrical system. To ward off such possibilities the second warring fluid is liberated. This chemical is cholinesterase. Its job is to annihilate the acetylcholine in the gap and thus break the connection. The entire war takes about 1/500 of a second. In other words the switch can be turned off and on 500 times each second.

THE UNDECIDED SWITCH

Poisons create any number of abnormal situations at the nerve/muscle junction. What if a poison prevented acetylcholine from ever getting across the gap? A substance like curare, the famous Indian arrow poison and modern medical muscle relaxant, is such a poison. It blocks the nerve signal to varying degrees, depending on the dosage. An overdose of curare can literally relax a body to death. It could paralyze the breathing apparatus and cause death by suffocation.

On the other hand we have the opposite effect. There are poisons like one called neostigmine which block or dampen

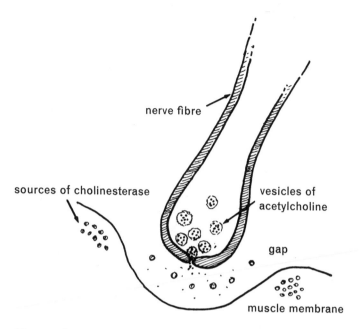

nerve fibre

sources of cholinesterase

vesicles of
acetylcholine

gap

muscle membrane

The gap between the nerve ending and the muscle is vulnerable to the effects of poison.

the action of the enzyme cholinesterase. This means that there is no way to destroy the acetylcholine in the gap and the build-up sets up short-circuit conditions. There would be continuous stimulation and the victim would (in extreme cases) die of over-excitation (observed as spasms and twitches).

Poisons act in a number of ways to approach one of these two extremes: over-relaxation and over-excitation.

Curare, just mentioned, for example interferes with the nerve junction's operation somewhat indirectly. It spreads its molecules in such a way that it coats the muscle membrane side of the gap. This simply blocks off the acetylcholine when it tries to attach itself to the surface.

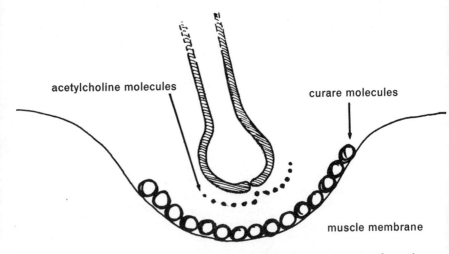

acetylcholine molecules

curare molecules

muscle membrane

Curare molecules block the action of acetylcholine in the nerve/muscle junction.

Botulin, the poison produced by the bacterium *Clostridium botulinum,* on the other hand, acts by preventing the release of acetylcholine in the first place. The net effect, however, is much the same. No signal gets through and the muscle relaxes— or collapses! Botulin, incidently, is such a powerful poison— sometimes claimed to be the most poisonous substance in the world—that a mere smidgen results in paralysis, suffocation and probably death.

In brief: *Monkey wrench number three* is the poison which keeps the signal from getting through or which distorts and changes its meaning. Most damage is caused by abnormal or closed-off switches—nerve/muscle junction points. One class of poisons which causes such abnormal operation of the body's control signals is the nerve poison. The number of nerve/muscle junctions can't compete with the number of molecules in a small amount of poison. A case of poisoning, more often than not, involves two or three of our particular "monkey wrenches." And it all adds up to destruction and death!

Adding It Up

Death by poisoning is seldom a simple process. Other general points to consider when judging the outcome of poisoning are:

The efficiency of the poisoning process.

How many molecules does it take to destroy key enzymes and vital body cells and fluids? How many are wasted and sidetracked?

The particular tissues and organs involved.

Some poisons do not kill directly. They may, for instance, cause the liver cells to disintegrate slowly. Death would follow not from the poison directly but from the side effects, which may develop over weeks or months. Sometimes there is a race between the destruction of cells and their normal regeneration by the organ involved.

The distribution of the poison.

Poisons tend to be unevenly distributed when absorbed. Some bind more strongly with body proteins, some with blood and some with nerve tissue. Certain poisons find it difficult to reach the brain and other parts of the nervous system. This is a result of the "blood-brain barrier." Fatty material surrounding the small capillaries of the nervous system tends to repel water and consequently any compound that happens to be dissolved in it. A water-soluble poison would thus have extra difficulty reaching the brain or spinal cord.

The state of the victim.

Health, sex, allergies, age, previous exposure level, emotional state and many other factors of one's past and present condition play some part, large or small, in the body's final battle with the poison.

The state of the animal.

Victims of snakebite, for example, receive venom of variable quality. It depends on the snake's size, age, "state of anger" and previous history.

The number of poisons involved.

Venoms have a variety of different poisons, each component poison doing something different. It is possible that adding poisons together may produce a lethal "one-two punch."

The way the poison is ingested.

Whether a poison is eaten, breathed in, injected under the skin, deep into a muscle or absorbed through the skin makes a great deal of difference. Certain venoms, for example, can be swallowed with no harmful results. If the same venom is injected into the blood death is immediate.

The Search for the Universal Antidote

There have always been attempts to discover a single antidote which would be effective against the entire range of poisonous plants, animals and minerals. For 2500 years dust filed from the precious horn of the unicorn was thought to protect against all deadly poisons. Today the best that science can offer is "activated charcoal." The question is, how good is it?

Back in 1830 or so a Parisian pharmacist by the name of P. F. Touery maintained that very finely powdered charcoal was the true universal antidote. To prove his theory he arose before members of the French Academy and, as they watched, he downed a massive dose of poison—ten times the lethal dose of the ugliest poison he could find. The poison was strychnine. He followed the poison with a charge of powdered charcoal, about 15 grams or half an ounce. The astonished audience saw him walk away without so much as a twitch (strychnine would have killed him by causing violent and uncontrollable convulsions). With this demonstration charcoal was "in" as the universal antidote. It held this position until World War I, when it was used as an absorbent in gas masks. Then it disappeared from the European scene.

Charcoal was used long before 1830 in other parts of the world. It was known, for example, to the South American Indians centuries ago. Historians write of Indian tribes inserting finely powdered and lightly warmed charcoal into the nostrils to stop nose bleeds. They also mention the use of "wood soot" in tea to soothe intestinal disorders, ashes from tobacco and mountain laurel to treat ulcers, and water poured over charcoal to cure sore throat and cough. No doubt these cures with charcoal had some basis in fact but their charcoal was not the "activated" charcoal used in the universal antidote recommended by physicians and pharmacists.

WHAT IS ACTIVATED CHARCOAL?

Activated charcoal looks like wood soot but has more remarkable (though invisible) powers. The secret is in the activation process itself.

Activated charcoal is made by an industrial process which involves the controlled heating of burned wood, peat, bone, nutshells, or coal. Temperature is held close to 1000°F (540°C) while an atmosphere of water vapor, carbon dioxide, or air covers the partly burned source materials. Processes vary in detail but they all somehow "activate" the final product. That is, they cause the formation of an enormous number of fine pores. As the fineness of a powder increases its surface increases proportionally. To illustrate this process, suppose we start with a piece of wood the size of a sugar cube and cut it into eight equal parts. The area exposed would double. If each of the resulting cubelets is cut into eight additional pieces the area will again double. After thousands upon thousands of such divisions the area resulting from the original cube becomes enormous. We see the final result in activated charcoal. It is these fine pores which collect the gases, liquids, or various dissolved substances in the host fluid (the strychnine dissolved in water, for instance). The pores are roughly a millionth of an inch in diameter. If the surface they create could be stretched out and measured it would come to about a thousand square feet (90 square metres) for one gram (.035 ounces) of charcoal. The graphite downed by Touery would have the area of a half dozen modern ranch style homes. This large absorption surface is what allows graphite to absorb its own weight in noxious materials. It is effective against virtually all poisons except cyanide, corrosives, strong alkalies (like drain opener) and strong mineral acids (like hydrochloric). The following table lists most of the substances absorbed by activated charcoal.

SUBSTANCES ABSORBED BY ACTIVATED CHARCOAL		
Alcohol	Iron	Phenolphthalein
Antimony	Mercuric chloride	Phosphorus
Antipyrene	Methylene blue	Potassium permanganate
Arsenic	Morphine	Quinine
Atropine	Muscarine	Salicylates
Barbiturates	Nicotine	Silver
Cantharides	Opium	Stramonium
Camphor	Oxalates	Strychnine
Cocaine	Parathion	Sulfonamides
Digitalis	Penicillin	Tin
Ipecac	Phenol	

To test the effectiveness of activated charcoal a lethal dose of poison was given to two groups of mice. One group was then given activated charcoal while the other wasn't. The result: all the mice receiving activated charcoal lived. Those in the other group were all dead within ten minutes.

The Hemodetoxifier

While poisons are within the stomach activated charcoal will be unusually effective. But once poison is absorbed into the blood it is beyond the reach of the charcoal. At least it was until the 1960's when Yatzidis Hippocrates showed that activated charcoal *could* absorb poisons from the blood. Today an instrument called the B-D Hemodetoxifier brings blood to the charcoal and permits the absorption of many poisons. The device has been successful in treating drug overdoses of amobarbital, chlordane, ethchlorvynol, glutihimide, metho-

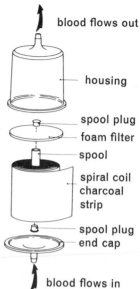

blood flows out

housing

spool plug

foam filter

spool

spiral coil charcoal strip

spool plug

end cap

blood flows in

The blood flows into the hemodetoxifier cylinder where it passes through a coiled filter of activated charcoal which removes the toxic substances.

trexate, methsuximide, phenobarbital, salicylate, secobarbital, either singly or in combination. There appears to be no reason why the device may not, one day, be used for all substances which adhere to activated charcoal.

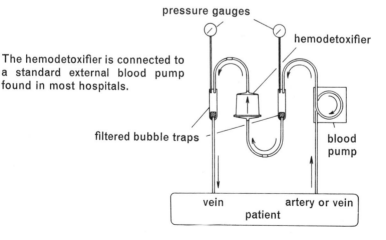

pressure gauges

hemodetoxifier

The hemodetoxifier is connected to a standard external blood pump found in most hospitals.

filtered bubble traps

blood pump

vein   artery or vein

patient

Exotic Poisons of Nature: Deadly Beasts of the World

> Each animal described in this chapter is strangely fascinating . . . exotic . . . for one reason or another. Altogether they represent the animal kingdom in the four corners of the world, a richness of past mythology and lore, and a present popularity in their own corner of the world (with but one exception)—all have one characteristic in common: they are intimately associated with an equally exotic super-poison.

Rattlesnake Country

Monsters past and present are pretty well represented by England's Werewolf, the Chinese Dragon and Romania's Vampire. A newcomer among monsters—the rattlesnake—was literally "made in America" and is as American as apple pie and tall tales from Texas.

WHAT MADE THE MYTHICAL MONSTER GROW?

The rattlesnake was imported from Europe some four hundred years ago and began its journey to monsterdom. It was in 1634 that a writer named Wood wrote that rattlers didn't kill with their breath (as was reported in England), nor did they sting, for the poison came from their teeth. Later a priest traveling in Canada wrote that rattlesnakes bite like dogs and inject venom through a small black sting. Then in 1877 another writer by the name of Dugees circulated the story that a rattlesnake leaves its venom glands on a rock when it goes to a stream or pond to drink. When it returns, if someone has stolen the venom glands in its absence, it dies in convulsions or kills itself by striking its head against the rocks.

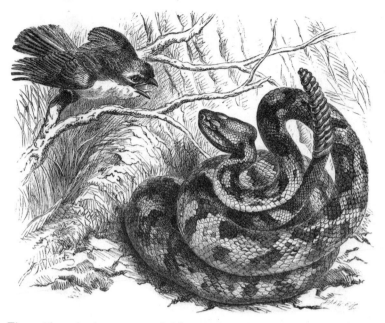

The rattlesnake is a successful hunter because he has the ability to sense the heat given off by small animals.

In 1931 Kincaid wrote in *The New Mexico Pastor* that he was informed by Mexican sheepherders that rattlers removed their fangs while courting, so as not to hurt each other. Also in the same year Thomas, in *Tall Stories*, came up with a whopper of a tale. He told about the rattler fleeing from a kingsnake so fast that the friction was setting the grass on fire, but that the trailing kingsnake was sweating so much in keeping up that it put out the fire. Their trail was a long, black streak through the grass.

Again in 1931 a writer named Boatright, in *Tall Stories from Texas*, wrote the yarn about the terrible tragedy of Peg-Leg Ike, who was bitten on his wooden leg and, despite the frantic efforts of friends armed with axes to chop away at the swelling timber, was choked to death by the fantastic growth. The sorrowful survivors, continued the tale, got enough kindling wood for the entire winter. In another story it was a sapling bit by a rattler. The sapling turned into a giant of a tree, the size of a California Sequoia.

It may only be a tall tale but there are some who believe a kingsnake, which has no poison fangs, can kill a rattler because it eats rattlesnake weed as an antidote to rattlesnake bite. The story goes that every time a rattler bites, the kingsnake hurries to a nearby snakeweed and nibbles off a leaf or two, then returns to the fight. The kingsnake is wise enough to always make sure the snakeweed is growing within easy reach. If the rattlesnake weed is not there the kingsnake will not fight the rattler.

Later, in 1934, Boatright added another topper. He told the story of a rattler and a kingsnake who swallowed each other up at the same time—they both naturally disappeared. His other stories were attributed to one Pecos Bill (said to be the West Texas cowpuncher's Paul Bunyan) and another Great Plains hero by the name of Febold Feboldson. Pecos Bill, it seemed, had it in for rattlers. He knew that rattlers eat moth balls but not chili powder. So he prepared some special moth balls with centers of mixed chili and nitroglycerine—but with the outside napthalene. When the coating melted off and the chili burned their insides, the rattlers struck their tails on rocks and exploded the nitroglycerine. Febold Feboldson, in yet another of Boatright's tales, is said to have owned a 14-foot rattler named Arabella. Once when Feboldson was tied up by Indians, Arabella squirted venom on the rope, and disintegrated it. On a stroll one day, Arabella rattled the snake's national anthem, and she and Feboldson were immediately surrounded by a huge assembly of her compatriots. Feboldson gave himself up for lost, but Arabella rattled Brahm's "Lullaby" and put her friends to sleep. Finally, in another story a farmer by the name of Frank Payne visited another farmer named Bill

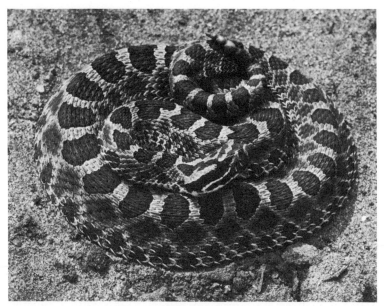

This ground rattlesnake (*Sistrurus catenatus*), measuring 12 inches (42.5 cm.) long was found near Great Bend, Kansas.

Mathes. On Mathes' farm in Galena, Missouri, Payne encountered a rattler which bit the handle of his hoe. In less than an hour it swelled up so big that they had to split it into four pieces, each as big as a railroad tie.

FALSE BELIEFS

Along with tall tales were the less outlandish claims which became common false beliefs. But they too fueled the growing image of the snake monster. For example: there was the belief that rattlers

- are real sports, giving the doomed one a head start before going after him
- bite with their teeth, then inject the venom from the branches of a forked tongue

- are vengeful—if a rattler loses a mate the other will get the killer, no matter what
- mesmerize their victims (they stare at the intended victim with an evil eye. If it happens to be a rabbit or bird the hypnotized creature will simply walk into the snake's wide-open mouth).

THE REAL MONSTER

Rattlers are cold-blooded creatures, which means that they tend to take on the temperature of their surroundings. For this reason they prefer 80 to 90°F (25 to 32°C). If it goes above 110°F (43°C) or below 50°F (10°C) they find it very hard to survive. In hot weather they prefer to be under the protection of large rocks; by day to be shielded from the sun and at night to receive the heat stored up during the day. In winter they hibernate, usually in a hibernaculum with hundreds of other snakes.

When they emerge from the winter's hibernation, usually in the month of May, they are anxious to prowl for food, preferably during warm nights and afternoons. This is the most dangerous time for man and snake to cross paths.

As hunters rattlers have several strikes against them. They are unimpressively slow movers on land, with a top speed of 3 miles (5 kilometres) per hour. They can, however, swim and climb trees quite well. They are pathetically nearsighted, limited to about 15 feet (4.5 metres). Further, they can't hear sounds. This would tend to cast doubt on the story in the 1937 Southwest Review, by a W. P. Webb, entitled *The Singing Snakes of the Karon Kawas*. In it Webb claims that he was told of the Indian who trained a band of rattlers to join him in song. With their rattlers they were able to carry four parts: soprano, alto, tenor and bass. True, rattlers don't hear sounds through the air but they are extraordinarily sensitive to vibrations coming through the ground. This, in fact, is one of the characteristics that make the rattler a good hunter.

The most unique characteristic, however, is his ability to see heat rays. The temperature-sensitive eye, located between the light-sensitive eye and the nose, enables him to distinguish between temperature differences of as little as a hundredth of a degree Fahrenheit (.02°C). To a rattler a mouse stands out from his surroundings like white against black, though the image is of heat rays rather than light rays. By the combined use of light, heat and vibration the rattler successfully stalks his intended victim.

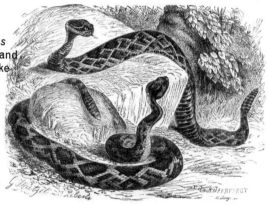

The eastern diamondback rattlesnake (*Crotalus adamanteus*) at top and the timber rattlesnake (*Crotalus horridus*) below.

At the fatal moment the rattler's claim to fame becomes obvious—that is, his striking power. It's been compared to a "short right to the bread basket" by the champ himself. High speed photography has shown the jab in slow motion. The jaws are open wide at the instant the head starts forward. In this same instant we see the retracted fangs in the upper jaw (normally positioned up, like the wheels in a flying airplane) instantly spring out. At the moment the jaw hits its target the mouth is wide open. Then the fangs sink in, muscles contract and venom is squeezed through the fangs. Finally the head is pulled back and the fangs snap back into place for another strike. All of this happens in the wink of an eye.

77

How does it feel to be bitten by a diamondback rattler? Herpetologist Gary Clarke was recently put through this private ordeal by poison. He was trying to weigh a large rattler called Big Red when disaster struck. (No matter how good the handler is, *no* snake will be compliant for very long.) Big Red was a 10-year-old, 52-inch, 6-pound rattler; the oldest, longest, and heaviest snake at the Midwest Research Laboratory in Kansas City, Missouri. In the autumn of 1959, Clarke was at work on scientific experiments involving some 30 snakes—including Big Red. "Weighing a snake can be tricky but the procedure is fairly simple," said Clarke. "Lift him out of the cage; drop him in a sack—generally a cotton flour sack; tie it in a knot and hang it on a balance scale. The snake's weight is the total minus the weight of the empty sack. The tricky part is how to release his head, take your hand away, and close the sack—in time to avoid getting bitten. You can't imagine how fast a snake can move. He'll be up before you can even blink. . . ." Clarke encountered difficulties and got off balance for just a moment—but that was long enough for Big Red to get out. "I felt a stab of pain in my left leg. His fangs were sunk into the underside of my knee. It happened so quickly, so unexpectedly." In a few moments, he reported, "My leg was on fire—it was like somebody was carving it up with red hot razor blades." Clarke applied first aid and one hour after the bite he was in the hospital. Then it got worse. "My leg began to swell, and every stretch exposed another nerve." About 11 hours after the bite he remarked: "Suddenly I felt an awful wave of nausea—and I vomited. Oh, I was sick, and completely out of control of any muscular contractions. Every heave was like a blowtorch on my leg." Immediate treatment, antitetanus and antivenin shots, 10 days of good hospital care, and *one other fact* saved Clarke from a worse fate: Big Red bit in a spot where it was impossible for him to close his fangs enough to inject a full dose.

From "Snake Bite" by Berton Rouché, *Today's Health*, December 1973, © The New Yorker, 1976.

Herpetologists (specialists in the field of reptiles) explain that rattler venom is like a "cocktail"—a potent mixture of some 25 ingredients. Although the venom hasn't as yet been completely analyzed chemically much can be said about its diabolical nature.

Rattler venom is more of a blood poison than a nerve poison. The venom, like all snake venoms, has 4 effects. It

- works on the nerves
- damages tissue in such a way that it spreads better
- digests and kills tissue
- causes much bleeding.

Venoms differ in detail. For example, the Eastern diamondback rattlesnake has a higher proportion of the digestive juices than do the other species. The Mojave rattlesnake has a higher proportion of the nerve component. All rattlesnake venoms have a considerable store of the bleeding factor. One of the main causes of death by rattlesnake bite is the result of suffocation, a lack of oxygen brought about by perforation of the blood vessels. Holes in the vessel walls allow blood to leak out so fast the heart can't circulate enough to keep up the vital supply of oxygen.

HISTORICAL ANTIDOTES

Antidotes have included songs, prayer, ritual dances, onions, garlic, herbs, gun powder, opium, vinegar, tobacco, kerosene and alcohol. Alcohol has always headed the list. In the days of the early American settlers few doctors failed to prescribe alcohol as a routine matter. Herpetologist Lawrence Klauber has collected several alcohol antidotes. Typical prescriptions included two quarts of corn whiskey every 12 hours; seven quarts of whiskey and brandy in four days; a quart of brandy the first hour, and another quart within two hours; one-half pint of bourbon every five minutes until a quart was consumed, and 104 ounces of applejack in four hours.

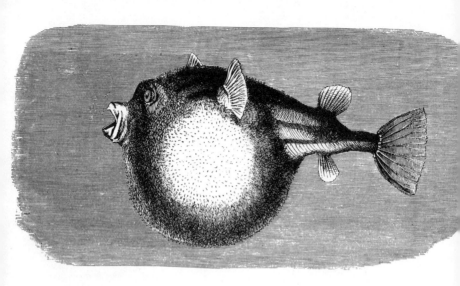

Puffers

Puffers (of the family Tetraodontidae) are best known for the famous fugu poison—virtually Japan's National Poison since it was first isolated there in 1950—and second best for the way they blow themselves into a ball and puff water when provoked or when searching for food at the bottom of the sea.

In Japan the puffer is known everywhere, and it has been for at least 1,500 years. In winter, when it tastes best (and is the most poisonous), it makes one of the land's supreme delicacies: fugu stew. Preparation of fugu stew is not only a matter of art and professional pride but of personal safety as well. That's why chefs and cooks must go to a special school to get a diploma in fugu stew preparation.

There are several reasons why such a diploma is called for.

- The poison, called tetrodoxin, is not weakened or destroyed by the heat of cooking.
- Only a trace—8 to 10 milligrams—is a fatal dose.
- The poison is not isolated in one organ but is found to some extent in all of the internal organs.

A most precise technique must be followed to get all traces out. In addition the removal must be accomplished within a certain time after the catch, before the poison begins to seep through to the meaty parts. The frequency of fugu poisoning is mute testimony to the difficulty of being a fugu stew expert. In one year there were 118 fatalities in 259 cases of poisoning. Death is always the result of paralysis of the breathing muscles and this in turn is caused by a depression of the respiratory center in the brain.

Scorpions

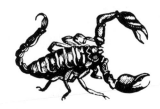

Scorpius the scorpion was recognized in the heavens as a constellation by the Babylonians of 2000 B.C. but it was the ancient Greeks to whom it owes its famous reign as the eighth house of the Zodiac. The Egyptian scorpion goddess, Selket, symbolized the good, for she had wings and held her arms high, as if to protect the mummies in their eternal quest. But then, at the same time, the scorpion was the symbol of the hangman.

The Bible has pictured the scorpion as a wretched, vicious beast associated with the black Judean wilderness and unbearable pain, for King Rehoboam said: "My father chastised you with whips, but I will chastise you with scorpions." Yet the scorpion is a creature kind enough to provide a cure for its own sting, for Pliny said: "It is thought good to lay to the sore the same scorpion that did the harm; or to eat him roasted, and last of all to drink it in two cups of pure wine of the grape."

On the other hand we find it hard to match the treachery of the scorpion and his hatred for the likes of man. Edward Topsell, the 17th century writer, tells of how scorpions got to a man sleeping on a raised bed in the middle of a room. They crawled on the ceiling and formed a chain hanging down over his bed, the last one down having the treat of stinging the unsuspecting sleeper. Aristotle countered this by mentioning a place called Carcia where scorpions are thoughtful enough never to sting a stranger—only the natives were ever stung.

The scorpion has eight grubby little legs, which makes it look more like a spider than the land animal it is. It has two large eyes and up to eight smaller ones on each side of its body—but it can't see. It has no teeth but it tears its victim to shreds with fang-like jaws. It is a desert animal but it seeks out caves and damp places. It injects venom with its tail—like a snake built backwards.

Scorpions play with victims as a cat does with a mouse, injecting venom and tearing the victim to shreds only if play gets out of hand. Prey includes grasshoppers, centipedes, worms, flies, beetles, spiders and, occasionally, younger scorpions. The scorpion table manners are nothing to speak of. As it eats its variety of victims it drools digestive juice over the victim or chunks of the victim. These partially digest the meat and make it into a liquid which is supped up. This takes considerable time, but when it's over the scorpion rolls up all the hard parts into a ball and leaves it as such.

During the day he hides under boards, in lumber and trash piles, under rocks or in loose dirt, but at night he comes out. Although he doesn't attack humans he often gets into shoes and clothing, causing indescribable commotion when he is found.

The Arizona Scorpion (*Centruroides sculpturatus*) is Arizona's most poisonous animal. It is abundant at the bottom of the Grand Canyon and especially in the vicinity of Phantom Ranch. The deadly species is about 8 inches (20 centimetres) long. Venom is produced in two glands at the end of its tail, both of which lead to the stinger at the very tip of the tail.

A sting is just an abrupt jab, over with in an instant.

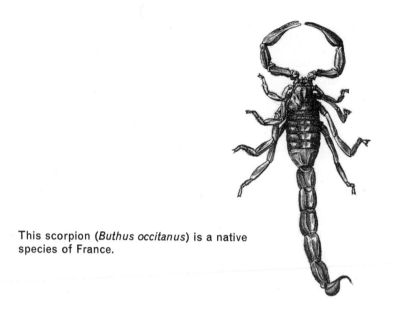

This scorpion (*Buthus occitanus*) is a native species of France.

Accuracy is amazing because the scorpion is segmented and therefore can move its body in any direction.

The sharp tip of the stinger makes a small wound which is spread apart by the conical stinger shaft. This puts the venom deep into the wound and allows the flesh to close back in over the wound. The bite of the deadly scorpion is hardly visible to the eye. Other species of scorpion produce wounds that swell, burn, and turn black and blue—but these are not the deadly types.

Scorpion venom is more poisonous, weight for weight, than snake venom. It has both a nerve poison to deaden sensations all over and another poison to act directly on the heart.

Symptoms include twitching and jerking, choking, blurred and otherwise disturbed vision and often fever as high as 103 or 104°F (39.5 or 40°C). Mild spasms have been known to come just before death. Fortunately scorpion antivenin is effective and available.

Gila Monster

The Gila monster is a big, slow and odd-looking lizard covered with a blanket of jet black and salmon pink glassy beads, somewhat in the pattern of a Navajo Indian blanket. The Gila's zoological name is *Heloderma suspectum*. Heloderma is another name for "nail-studded skin" and "suspectum" was chosen because for a long time it was only suspected that

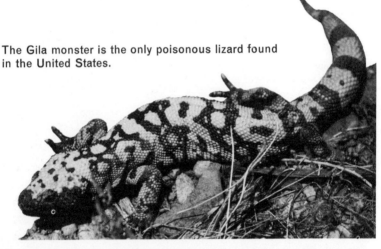

The Gila monster is the only poisonous lizard found in the United States.

he was poisonous. True, legends and tales had him spitting and blowing out venom, issuing forth a poisonous breath and coming on like a fiery dragon, but it was not known by more authoritative circles whether or not he really was poisonous. Today we know for sure. He is one of the two venomous species of lizard in North America (the other is the Mexican beaded lizard).

Victims of the Gila monster's bite are not as concerned about the deadliness of his venom as they are about the question of whether he will ever let go. It is no legend that the Gila "snaps like a turtle but holds on like a bulldog." Gilas, like turtles, do not lunge at a victim, but once his 35 teeth all sink in it will soon be over. The Gila has the monstrous habit of patiently holding the victim, occasionally grinding and chewing to work the poison in.

The tail of the Gila is something nearly everyone notices— especially if the hunting (or feeding) was bountiful. In the wild, when eggs from ground nesting birds, rabbits and quail are abundant, the Gila will store all the excess food in his tail, which assumes gigantic proportions. If his tail seems almost like that of a normal lizard we can be quite sure it's been a long while since his last banquet.

Cleopatra and the Asp

Serpents have always had the wisdom of the gods, for their weaving, undulating motion follows the waves of the sea and the sea embraces all of life's secrets and mysteries. This is a traditional belief in India. In fact, the father of Indian astronomy, whose name was Garga, was believed to owe all his knowledge to a snake. Then too, in India the cobra is believed to have the power of assuming the forms of gods, goddesses or messengers and two days a year—one in May and one in October—are set aside for his honor. The Hindus additionally set aside temples for Naja (Sanskrit for snake) and ascribe almost endless powers to him.

Looking at the cobra through less reverent eyes we see a fearsome beast, reaching up to 18 feet (5.4 metres) in length. He has a head the size of a boxer's hand and enough stored venom to dispatch 30 humans at once. The hood of the angered cobra adds a new dimension to snakedom, and especially so when we see him lean forward and sway to and fro as he threatens to strike. Even worse, he has a spine-chilling hiss and beady bronze eyes that seem to hypnotize the victim and prepare him for doom.

There's a story which appeared in an old English newspaper that recounts the snake's supposed hypnotic powers. A cobra raised his head and hissed at a hawk that had flown close by. The hawk gave a shriek and flapped its wings frantically to get away, but no amount of flapping would do. The evil eye of the cobra was more than a match for the sharp eye of the hawk and the hawk remained as if suspended in mid-air. In a few moments it was all over and the hawk plummeted down to his death.

Magnificent though his powers are, the king cobra does not have the greatest hood of all, nor is he the liveliest of the cobras. This distinction belongs to the 6 foot (1.8 metre) Egyptian cobra—the type used by the snake charmers. There's an unwritten law among cobra charmers that the snake they use must be full of life and deadly, not a dispirited mild type.

Snake charming is an old and noble profession. As often as not the charmer is a beautiful girl. In her act she grabs the snake behind the head with one hand and quick as a wink moves the other hand a safe distance in front of the snake. At the same moment she begins to move her hand to and fro, rhythmically. She is now depending on the snake's sharp eyesight, for the snake instinctively follows her hand and it all seems as if the snake is hypnotized and securely under her spell. The act usually ends by her kneeling very low and kissing the snake on its snoot. Sometimes Indian snake charmers play the flute and create the illusion that the snake dances to the tune of the flute. Not so, of course, for the cobra can't hear sounds. It is merely following the motion of the flute. Snake charming is somewhat less dangerous than it seems, for snake charmers

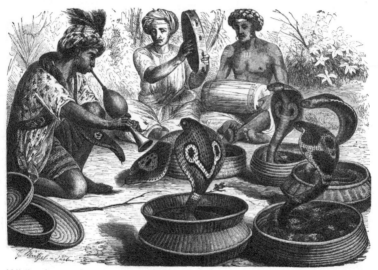

While the snakes appear entranced by the charmer's music, they are actually following the movement of the flute.

know exactly what the striking distance of their pet is. Usually this is between a fifth and a third of the overall length, or about 2 feet (60 centimetres). As young excitable cobras lash out to half their body length, good insurance would allow a little more than 2 feet.

It was Shakespeare who made the Egyptian cobra (also called an asp or worm) famous through the death scene of

Cleopatra. While captive in a monument in the city of Alexandria the great Egyptian Queen Cleopatra committed suicide by the "bite of the Asp." In 30 B.C. the war between Egypt and Rome finally ended and the Romans came to Egypt. The last of the Egyptian queens had done all she could for her country. She used her charms to win over two of the Roman conquerors but when Augustus Caesar came to Alexandria her luck ended because Augustus had no feeling for her charms and beauty. He spared her life but only so that he could make her march in his Parade of Triumph, as a common spoil of war. When Cleopatra learned of his intentions she committed suicide by having cobras smuggled into her place of captivity in the Alexandria monument.

> Cleopatra held the common belief that the angrier the cobra, the deadlier the venom. At least, that is, according to Shakespeare, whose Egyptian queen taunts the asp in order to arouse his anger and increase his venom's potency.
> "With thy sharp teeth this knot intrinsicate
> of life at once untie; poor venomous fool,
> Be angry, and dispatch. . . ."
> (*Antony and Cleopatra, Act V, Scene II*)
> The fact is that the snake's emotions do not affect the strength of the venom. However, the snake may bite down harder when angry, injecting the venom more deeply and speeding its deadly effect.

The bite of a cobra can kill an adult in fifteen minutes. More often though the victim becomes ill after ten minutes. Then in three hours he will have fuzzy vision, dizziness and slowed reflexes. The wound itself will be a little swollen. And in four to five hours breathing becomes like a heavy chore and in severe cases the victim just quits breathing.

Cobra venom is a nerve poison, three drops of which are deadly. On the scale of toxicity, weight for weight, it is 40 times as deadly as cyanide, 7 times more deadly than poisonous mushrooms, 5 times more deadly than the venom

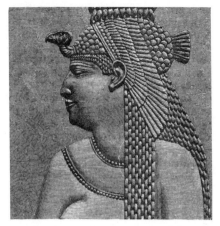

Cleopatra (69–30 B.C.), probably history's most famous snakebite victim.

of the black widow spider and about the same toxicity as scorpion venom.

Cobra venom has the one-two punch effect. Not only is it a number one nerve poison, but it has a factor (called lecithinase) which destroys red blood cells and another factor which paralyzes muscles directly, without bothering to go through the central nervous system first.

The Black Widow and the Red Back Spiders

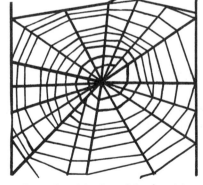

There's the popular notion that the black widow spider seizes her mate with voracious fangs and devours him right after their act of love, which is where the "widow" part of her common name came from. Being anywhere from ten to a hundred times the size of her mate she surely has the choice to eat or not to eat. The truth of the matter is that if food is not too scarce and if she feels content enough after the meeting she rarely chooses to eat him. More often than not he remains on her web and passes on after a few days, apparently from some sort of accelerated aging process. No matter—instinct makes the male spider eternally cautious. As he approaches her web he inches up slowly to where she is, then he destroys part of the web and isolates her to one small spot. Having done this he tries to touch her, and if she allows he will stroke her. Then he spins a fine web of silk all around her called the "bridal veil." After several hours in the web he finds conditions just right and spends the necessary five minutes or so with her. Then comes the fatal moment when she decides whether to eat him or let him be.

"Will you walk into my parlour? said the spider to the fly" is a saying that suggests that the spider is an evil archdemon full of intrigue and black virtue. The black widow has such a reputation for aggressiveness that she has been pictured as the Deviless spiriting after a Christian Soul. Nothing could be farther from the truth. The black widow is, in fact, a secretive sort of spinner, preferring to spin her web under rocks, between rocks, in trash piles, lumber piles, shady places near the ground and, as long as the old fashioned outdoor latrines exist, right under the essential devices. Reliable sources have it that in World War II so many soldiers were bitten that the antidote had to become a standard part of the medical kit. The fact is that anything whatever that touches her web suggests the possibility of a fly. Since her eyesight is nothing to speak of she uses the "logical deduction" that vibrations on the web mean "fly." Her zoological name is *Latrodectus mactans*: the first part, Latrodectus, was given because it so well described her real nature. It means "secret biter."

Black widow venom has four main poisons, three of which are deadly for insects. One part of the venom is what is called a stun poison. It acts fast, holding the victim until the slower poisons can do their job. Two other poisons damage the nervous system and later kill the stunned victim. The fourth poison is the well known nerve/muscle junction poison, effective against man and his kind. It poisons the nerve endings by keeping the nerve transmission fluid acetylcholine flowing until its supply is exhausted. This causes paralysis, eventually.

What does it feel like to be bitten by a black widow? Those who know say that it feels like the sting of a sharp needle. As the bite reddens (in moments) it begins to throb and pain begins to spread toward the center of the body. First the thighs, then the shoulders and back become painful. Next the stomach region becomes "stiff as a board." Weakness and trembling follow this. The pulse weakens, the skin becomes clammy, the breathing difficult and the mind dulled. Shock and paralysis follow in the more extreme cases. The whole sequence will be over in two or three days—for better or worse.

Spiders live by their juice too. They secrete compounds other than venoms. As they have no jaws for chewing they puncture their prey, inject digestive juices and wait till its insides become fluidlike. Then they merely sup it up.

The black widow has developed a trade-mark, possibly a warning device, that goes along with her jet black body—the famous red-orange hourglass on her belly.

The red back spider is Australia's answer to the American black widow and the New Zealand katipo. The "little animals" are almost identical in every way. In place of the hourglass on the underbelly of the American black widow the Australian red back has a red stripe. She is not identical to the black widow but the resemblance is remarkable. She's a satiny black spider who spins a messy web, is deadlier than the male and about six times as large, and (it is said) eats her mate too.

Stonefishes

Stonefishes are *the* most venomous fish known to man—and their delivery system is one of a kind too. Thirteen or 14 *very* sharp spines on their backs are fed from small sacs of venom on either side of the spine. The sacs are located beneath the skin. The slightest pressure imaginable causes poison to flow up the spine grooves to the point of contact. If several of these sharp spines manage to puncture the skin they introduce a most deadly nerve poison into the victim. There is terrible pain and cases have been reported where death followed in only two hours. More often it is four hours. If the victim lives as long as six hours after the puncture his chances for life are good, but there are still problems. The excruciating pain may drive him to insanity, and if he survives the pain his arms and legs may swell to enormous proportions for days or weeks. Finally, nausea may plague the victim for a year or more afterward.

The stonefish poison is supposed to exist in the interests of his own self-defense only, but in view of the record it would hardly seem so, for this ugly fish that looks like a rock can also lie as still as one. Moreover, it insists on lying about in shallow waters frequented by swimmers and waders. No matter how closely the swimmers may look, stonefish camouflage is so perfect that they could be looking right at him and never realize it. If the swimmer is lucky he will contact only a few of the spines. If he steps heavily enough to contact all 13 or 14, heaven help him then!

Stonefishes are quite widespread. They are found all along the shores of the Indian Ocean and the Western Pacific and all the way up to the Red Sea and down to Australia.

Natives have used their own antidotes for a long time (a scientific antidote *is* available today). Shredded papaya has been put on the sting sites to relieve the pain (as meat tenderizers like papaya juice have been known to do for other kinds

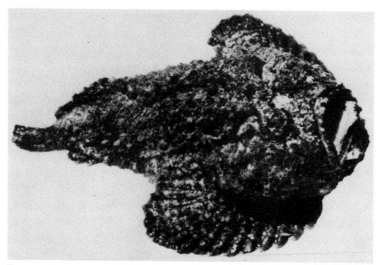

The most venomous fish in the world, the stonefish, is nearly invisible in its natural setting.

of stings). A popular remedy with the natives is to cut the gall bladder from a stonefish, extract it in water and swallow the extract. No reason for its success can be offered but the natives believe in it.

The Taipan

From the remote coastal regions of northern Australia and New Guinea comes the taipan, Australia's biggest, most poisonous and most dangerous snake; certainly one of the cleverest snakes in the whole world.

He attacks man and beast like no other snake does.

The taipan's extremely well developed sense of smell and his good eyesight allow him to track down, strike and immobilize his bestial victim. If it also happens to be his favorite food—the rat—he will swallow the creature whole. Australia, it seems, has a rat problem. The sugar cane fields are wonderful attractants and so the rat population skyrockets around sugar cane farms especially. As the rat is the taipan's favorite food, the taipan population tends to build up too. (The farmers have a gruesome choice unless they come up with a better solution for rat control.) The taipan is known to go down a rat hole and strike in succession with such speed that the entire rat population is dead in moments. The fearsome snake locates rats by his sense of smell, follows their movements with his good eyesight and then strikes with a hard-to-match rapidity. The rats never have a chance.

Snakes do have a sense of smell normally but the taipan's is extraordinarily well developed. What makes it super is the fact that he can "taste air" so well. This is what all snakes do when they flick their forked tongues back and forth. The tongue picks up odor particles from the air and then whips them back to a special organ located on the roof of the mouth.

Taipans are retiring, timid creatures. They won't attack a human unless cornered or startled, but when they do there is a certain viciousness that is hard to figure out. He flattens his head and neck straight up and raises part of the forebody up off the ground. At the same time the tail is raised up, weaving to and fro. After a few moments of this entrancing gyration he strikes—not once like other snakes do, but as a quick series of three or four snaps. The victim has no chance because most of the venom is delivered in the first one or two strikes and, by the time the victim knows what has happened, an extra one or two snaps have been made beyond what was needed.

An Australian farmer at Mossman years ago blamed a taipan living in the hollow of an old mango tree on his property for the loss of certain stock. The farmer went to kill the snake with a hoe, but the taipan was too fast for the farmer and his hoe. The farmer was bitten, ran to his house nearby and died there almost immediately. There has *never* been a definite case of taipan bite which has not been fatal to the human victim.

94

Taipan venom is not only potent but the amount injected is always far, far more than enough. Eric Worrell of the Australian Reptile Park near Gosford, where taipans are milked for venom research, calculated that the taipan's stock of venom could kill 23,500 laboratory mice.

The bite of the taipan (*Oxyuranus scutellatus*) gives all the symptoms of deep intoxication. The venom tends to destroy red blood cells. That is, it would were it not that it also paralyzes the central nervous system which causes breathing to stop . . . and death!

The Ultimate Bug

For many years it was believed that poison (toxin) from the bacterium *Clostridium botulinum* was the most powerful in the world. It's seven million times more potent than cobra venom and one ounce (properly distributed) could wipe out everyone in the United States. Yet there is room for debate about records. The Military has a substance in their biological warfare arsenal that they call Q-fever. It is so powerful that one ounce could wipe out 30 billion people, everyone in the world seven times over. They also have a weapon called "Dengue Fever" which is so powerful that *one* organism, less than a trillionth of a gram, could cause death. This raises the question: Is it proper to call one organism a "lethal dose?" After all, it isn't the one lone organism that causes death, but rather the poisons produced by the millions upon millions of organisms that multiply in the body of the victim. The argument still stands—but considering the consequences there is not too much wrong with calling "Organism #1" a "lethal dose."

The bacterium causing botulism lurks in all the earth's soil and is of harm to no one until very unusual conditions happen to arise. With do-it-yourself canning and preserving on the rise botulism takes on a new sense of importance. In one instance a housewife died by tasting only part of a cold green bean from a spoiled jar.

Symptoms appear only after several hours, for the poison is slow in absorption. But once it reaches the blood stream a rapid succession of symptoms appear: seeing double, drooping eyelids, a very tired feeling, dizziness, difficulty in swallowing and—finally—death by paralysis of the muscles that control breathing.

The poison attaches itself to the nerve endings that join to the muscles and somehow interferes with the production of the nerve transmission fluid called acetylcholine. This means that fewer and fewer impulses reach the muscles and paralysis creeps in, first of the muscles of the eye, nose and throat, then the breathing muscles.

Where does the bug come from?

The tiny bugs of botulism seem to have avoided the evolutionary ladder—they haven't changed in form much for 2,000,000,000 years. In the world at that time there was no oxygen to speak of and life forms that preferred such an atmosphere flourished. Some time later green plants started to evolve and put oxygen into the atmosphere. They have flourished since that time and living things that prefer our present kind of atmosphere have prospered. Those that were sensitive to oxygen tended to die or develop ways of resisting. The bacterium of botulism went into suspended animation by developing a thick resistant coating around itself—it became a "spore." In this condition it can lie in the soil and exist almost indefinitely, in drought, temperatures ranging between absolute zero (minus 459°F or minus 273°C) to the temperature of boiling water (212°F or 100°C).

Spores exist nearly everywhere, so they always find their way into a jar at canning time. If they aren't killed by proper heating they remain inside until some mysterious sense tells the spore to come out of its coating and take advantage of the primordial conditions of botulin paradise, just as it was

2,000,000,000 years ago. There is plenty of food, the temperature isn't too bad and there is no oxygen again (assuming a good job of vacuum packing was done). These ideal conditions coax the production of toxins, something which the bacteria didn't do while in the soil outside.

In brief: For its paradise the bacterium of botulism needs a total lack of oxygen (even touching air for an instant will destroy it); any temperature between absolute zero and that of boiling water (ten minutes in a pressure cooker at 250°F or 121°C kill the spores); proteinaceous foods, such as beans and fish; and a mildly alkaline fluid medium (usually found in green beans but not canned tomatoes: any acid condition will darken the paradise). The toxin, once produced, is destroyed by cooking. The housewife died because she tasted a *cold* green bean straight from the jar. The most infamous botulism deaths in recent years occurred when people ate poorly packaged vichyssoise, a soup which is served cold.

All told there are five types of botulism, each linked to a different kind of food: types A, B, C, D and E. Types A and B come from meats and fruits, type C from birds, and types D and E from fish. Botulism was first discovered in Germany in 1735 and was associated with sausage. (The disease was named for this sausage: "botulus" is Latin for sausage.) Type A was first identified in 1895 and Type E as recently as 1951. Since botulism comes in types, the antidote is "polyvalent," aimed at all the possible strains at once. Its effect can't be certain because the antidote is a catch-all device and is not designed for guaranteed results.

The Vampire

Bats are unearthly creatures that dart about in the warm, still summer evening and inspire eerie thoughts. These are the weird creatures with the face of Old Nick the Devil himself and who refuse to identify with any other kind of animal. And among the bats the vampire has the worst reputation of all.

In 1897 Bram Stoker wrote the now classic novel *Dracula*, and put the vampire in a new and peculiar light. Moviegoers since 1931 have seen the shady Count Dracula spread his huge cape and transform into a vampire bat before their very eyes. The vampire according to legend was the soul of a dead person which at night took the form of a bat and searched about the countryside for a victim from whom to suck blood. Dracula's Romania had bats, of course, but the idea of *bloodsucking* bats was imported from America. Around 1725 explorers came to Central and South America and actually encountered huge bats, with wing spreads of 15 inches (37 centimetres). When they returned to Europe we can imagine how the stories began to grow.

The vampire bat, dubbed also *Desmodus rotundus*, is a true vampire: It lives *only* on the blood of mammals. It also has the reputation of being such a glutton that it drinks blood until it's so round that it could roll like a ball. The 4 to 5 tablespoons (60 to 75 millilitres) it drinks each night comes to about 5 gallons (19 litres) a year.

The vampire's whole being seems dedicated to the task of stealing blood. Two sharp, elongated front teeth are ideal for snipping out a small section of skin and making a trough for the oozing blood to fill. Then the long tongue is used to sup out the blood, as through a straw and unlike the lapping of a dog or cat. The V-shaped groove in its lower lip is used to shape the tongue into a rounded form. And to keep the wound agitated and the blood flowing the tongue darts in and out like a small piston.

Yet the vampire manages to do all this without inflicting pain. It seems that without effort at all it can light on a victim, gouge out a small bit on his nose or toe, gorge itself and be off. In the morning the victim will be shocked and surprised to find the wound often still oozing blood. No wonder myths

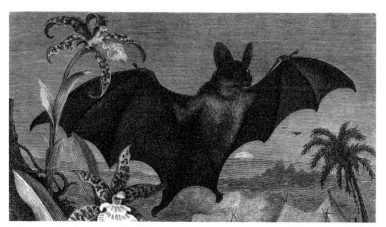
The dreaded vampire bat.

used to picture a hypnotic emanation coming from the bat's wings as it fluttered silently over its victim.

Leo E. Miller, while in British Guiana, described his experience with a vampire one night. He decided to lay awake and catch a vampire he saw in his room. After a while he heard a flutter in the darkness. Then something struck the covers some distance from his exposed feet. He could feel the bat slowly work its way up the sheets until it reached his foot. Suddenly he struck at it and missed. The bat fluttered around the room a bit, out of the way, until all was quiet again. Then the whole scene was replayed several times. Finally Miller dozed off a few minutes and awoke to find that the stealthy bat was successful.

Bats have the uncanny knack of knowing just when the victim is asleep. At that moment they alight close by and walk deliberately up to the point of attack.

True, the vampire raises shudders and drinks blood but it's not the blood we lose that matters so much. Rather it's the infinitesimally minute amount of poison producer that we gain from the bite: that is, the deadly virus of paralytic rabies, the hydrophobia of the mad dog. The poison produced by this virus is always deadly . . . if we fail to get the antidote/treatment in time. Vampires themselves don't often suffer from the disease but they transmit it nonetheless. The bite of a bat is considered rabid unless *proven* otherwise by lab tests.

RABIES

What causes rabies? The disease is caused by a virus which attacks the nervous system. Virus from the bite of the bat travels from the wound to the brain where it multiplies in the brain cells and then spreads to other parts of the body. Symptoms usually start in one or two months and last from several days to three weeks. At first there is restlessness and depression. This is followed by anxiety and a growing fear which mounts into terror and uncontrollable rage. (This is caused by the irritation of brain cells.) In a matter of some days the damage deepens and extreme sensitivity follows. The mere pressure of a light breeze brings excruciating pain. Following this muscle spasms begin. There is so much pain in swallowing that no liquids can be taken and the victim becomes as dehydrated as if he were in the desert. There is a great dread of strangling and the mere mention of water or thought of swallowing makes a raging maniac of the victim. Finally death follows as the breathing muscles are paralyzed.

Is there a cure? Well, by some miracle, two (very difficult) cures have been recorded, but based on the fact that in 1975 nearly 7,000 people worldwide died of rabies (from skunks, foxes, dogs, raccoons and bats) the odds are poor. Well over a million Americans are bitten by animals each year and out of this number 30,000 undergo the rather painful treatment for cases of suspected rabies.

The treatment involves 21 injections of rabies-vaccine booster shots and one serum-immune globuline injection. The injections are given every day—with the treatment spread over several weeks.

Borgias Among the Bufos

A giant three-pound tropical night-feeding toad called *Bufo marinus* is an unusual combination of professional killer and garbage disposal unit. Bufo (for short) came from South America in the 1930's, stayed over for a few years in Hawaii and was drafted from Hawaii into the Australian service, where his task was to rid the fields of the voracious sugar cane beetle. He devoured the hated beetle but soon took to doing the same with cabbages, table tennis balls, loads of other insects, and other toads. In addition he poisoned dogs, cats and cattle. But it wasn't his insatiable appetite alone that made him into the world's worst toad and a national calamity for Australia. It was the fact that Mrs. Bufo laid upwards of 40,000 eggs each year.

Once the Bufos were confined to Queensland in the northeast of Australia by the forbiddingly dry and hot natural surroundings, thought to be as effective for toads as the moat around a castle for the knights of old. Not so. A few escaped and caused great alarm. In the wet season, explained an Australian reptile expert, they could get into the river pools (and other bodies of water) and multiply so fast that they would force out the native species, create an "evolution explosion" and run amuck to other regions of Australia. The Wild Life Department and Darwin Conservation Society planned an offensive against the few escapees. Thirty dollars a piece was the going reward. There were WANTED: DEAD OR ALIVE signs posted and a radio station broadcast the mating call to lure the females out of hiding.

Bufo, incidentally, is a toad—not a frog. The frog is a moist, relatively smooth-skinned fellow with an enormous capability for jumping. A toad, on the other hand, is a clumsy creature covered by a rough, dry, warty skin. His reputation is none too good either. In common folklore he was believed to carry his heart in his neck, possess two livers and possess both poisons and a demonic spirit. And in *Paradise Lost* John Milton had Satan take the form of a toad and inject poison into the sleeping Eve's ear.

Bufos secrete a poisonous fluid from a pair of glands located behind their eyes. The fluid was found to have 25 different components. A major part was bufagin, a heart stimulant similar to the digitalis of the foxglove plant. Another was cinobufagin, an anesthetic affecting nerve endings (the anesthetic is said to be 90 times as powerful as the narcotic cocaine). A nerve poison, resembling the muscle relaxant curare, is also present. A victim of the Bufo poison suffers nausea, throwing up, high blood pressure, headaches and paralysis. In one experiment an extract from the Bufo glands was given to snakes. First, to non-toad-eating snakes. Three milligrams caused "heart failure" in the snakes. Three times this dosage caused "heart failure" in "veteran" toad-eating snakes.

"KOKOI"

Bufo poisons may soon be used to duplicate or improve an old Chinese remedy made of dried toad skins, a concoction called Ch'an Su. It has been used for millennia to cure sores, toothaches and sinus conditions. The effects Bufo poisons have on Australian dogs, cats and cattle are only too well known but its effects on man can only be guessed at through the poison arrows used by the Cholo Indians of western Colombia.

The poison they use is called *Kokoi*. It comes from Bufo's smaller Central and South American relatives. These are small brightly colored frogs (*Dendrobates phyllobates*) that inhabit the steaming hot jungles. These frogs produce a poisonous compound called batrachotoxia which kills its victims by permanently blocking the transmission of nerve signals to the muscles. It is said to be ten times as effective as tetrodoxin, the fugu poison mentioned in the novel *Dr. No*.

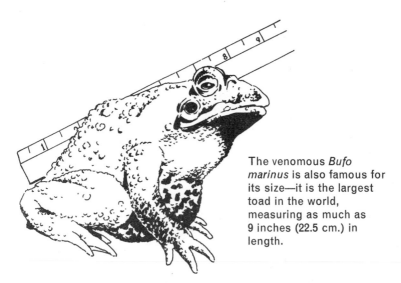

The venomous *Bufo marinus* is also famous for its size—it is the largest toad in the world, measuring as much as 9 inches (22.5 cm.) in length.

One frog skin can furnish one milligram, which is enough to poison 50 darts and kill 50 men.

To prepare a poison arrow (or dart) the Indians impale a frog on a spit of wood, then roast it alive over an open fire until heat causes pain and the frog cries. (Pain is the only reason a frog exudes its poison: the frog, in effect "cries.") Soon the poison bubbles up, as blisters form on the skin. Arrow tips are prepared by touching them to the skin, or the venom can be allowed to drip out of the skin glands to be caught in some sort of natural container and allowed to ferment. Arrow tips dipped in either form drop monkeys and birds in their tracks. Nerve paralysis is almost instantaneous.

South American Indians use the chemical called bufotenine (from the skins of poisonous toads). It is also employed in their cohoba snuff (*Piptadenia peregrina*) to promote a feeling of well-being when they hold dances. In larger doses cohoba snuff induces trances during which the Indians speak with their gods and the Spirits of their dead.

103

The Infamous Shellfish

There's an old wives' tale well taken to heart by fishermen and their clans about not eating shellfish during a month with a missing R. Modern biologists tell us its a pretty good idea. Here's why.

During the warm months of the year there's a species of plankton that drifts and floats on the sea like so much flotsam and jetsam. These plankton, called *Gonyaulaux catenella* (also marine dinoflagellate), are strange little creatures about as big as a microbe that by the millions make up the menu of the various shellfish: oysters, scallops, clams and mollusks. During the warm months the plankton secrete a poison known as saxitoxin and the shellfish eat both plankton and poison.

The saxitoxin gathered up and concentrated by the shellfish was first extracted from them by scientists to help develop a good test for the presence of poisonous saxitoxin in shellfish headed for market, and to help create new and useful drugs. After the Central Intelligence Agency took an interest in saxitoxin a better extraction method was apparently found. Nonetheless, we are told by government workers that it takes literally thousands of the large Alaskan Butter Clams (about 100 pounds or 45 kilograms) to yield a mere gram (the weight of about 25 drops of water).

Saxitoxin was first intended to replace the "Cyanide L-pill" issued to American agents in World War II. It never really found its way into the cloak and dagger arena, though it was used as the poison in the silver dollar carried by U-2 pilot Gary Powers in his flight over the USSR in 1960. Saxitoxin was put into the grooves of a tiny pin hidden in the silver dollar. The pin was to be used in the event of capture. As it turned out the Russians seized the silver dollar, found the concealed pin, and out of curiosity tried its power out on one of their huge guard dogs . . . which was dead 10 seconds later!

Exotic Poisons of Nature: Poisonous Plants of the World

Poison gardens are easy to plant. A spacious home yard might include plants such as the following: castor bean, daffodil, hyacinth, aconite, lily-of-the-valley, foxglove, English ivy, oleander, wisteria, yew, wild cherry, elderberry, chinaberry, death camas, jimson weed, hemlock and the nightshades. And around Christmas: holly, mistletoe and poinsettia. An array such as this would make a fit rival for the legendary home garden of the Sorceress Medea, set up for her by the Kings in the mythical Kingdom of Colchius and guarded by walls "nine fathoms deep." Inside grew poisons and antidotes, side by side. A few of Medea's favorites, such as henbane, belladonna and aconite are covered in what follows—as are other strangely different and fascinating—exotic—poisons.

Socrates and the Cup of Hemlock

Hemlock reaches far back into history. Of all the poisonous plants known to the ancient Greeks none could rival hemlock. The Greeks used it to make their exit from this world, for, if committed according to the proper rules and rituals, suicide was a respectable way to go. Hemlock was also the Athenian State Poison and "the cup of Hemlock" was used in State executions. The Executioner himself was required to oversee the preparation of the fateful brew and to ensure its potency.

Probably the most famous execution of all time was that of the ancient Greek philosopher Socrates. He was sentenced to die "by the cup" in 402 B.C. for corrupting the minds of Athenian youth. An intimate description is given by his long-time disciple and former student, Plato.

"When the fatal cup was brought he asked what it was necessary for him to do. 'Nothing more,' replied the servant of the judges, 'than as soon as you have drunk the draught, to walk about until you find your legs become weary and afterwards lie down upon your bed.'

"He took the cup without any emotion or change in his countenance and, looking at him in a steady and assured manner,

" 'Well!' said he, 'what say you of this drink?'

" 'May a libation be made out of it?'

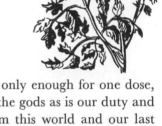

Poison hemlock (*Conium maculatum*).

"Upon being told that there was only enough for one dose, 'At least,' said he, 'we may pray to the gods as is our duty and implore them to make our exit from this world and our last stage happy, which is what I most ardently beg of them.'

"Having spoken these words he remained silent for some time and then drank off the whole draught.

"After reproving his friends for indulging in loud lamentations, he continued to walk about as he had been directed until he found his legs grow weary. Then he lay down upon his back and the person who had administered the poison went up to him and examined for a little time his feet and legs, and then squeezing his foot strongly, asked whether he felt him? Socrates replied that he did not. He then did the same to his legs, and proceeding upwards in this way, showed us that he

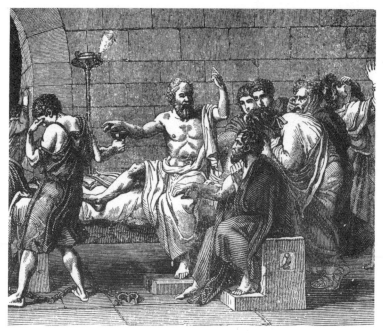
Socrates, surrounded by his disciples, takes the fatal cup.

was cold and stiff, and he afterwards approached him and said
to us that when the effect of the poison reached the heart
Socrates would depart. And now the lower parts of his body
were cold, when he uncovered himself and said, which were
his last words, 'Crito, we owe Aesculapius a cock. Pay the
debt and do not forget it.'

" 'It shall be done,' replied Crito. 'But consider whether you
have anything else to say.'

"Socrates answered in the negative, but was in a short time
convulsed. The man then uncovered him; his eyes were fixed
and when Crito observed this he closed his eyelids and his
mouth."

Death by the cup of hemlock comes in a strange way. There

is creeping coldness and paralysis which is keenly felt and experienced—but the mind is totally helpless when it tries to respond. Coldness and death move in stages, from the feet upwards. First the legs become numb, then the feet and arms become cold and the cold moves slowly to the brain. Death occurs when the muscles which control breathing become paralyzed, following depression of the controlling function in the brain. The account of Socrates' death shows this sequence. Socrates' mind is clear to the very end which occurs moments after he asks about the sacrifice to Aesculapius (the god of the Medical Arts). It was only by analyzing Socrates' symptoms that historians could conclude that the plant used was actually poison hemlock (that is *Conium maculatum*) and not water hemlock (*Cicuta maculatum*). Both are closely related in every way except in the symptoms they produce. Water hemlock produces violent convulsions instead of muscle paralysis as Socrates experienced. Moreover the historians found records which showed that poison hemlock actually grew in Greece and particularly in the vicinity of Athens. It all added up and they concluded that Socrates died by the cup of (poison) hemlock. In the time of Socrates it was referred to as "Cicuta," according to the Roman scholar Pliny. The word "hemlock" is a 10th century Anglo-Saxon expression which combines their word for shore ("hem") with the word "leac." The scientific name (*Conium maculatum*) was provided by the father of classification, Linnaeus, only as recently as 1737.

Poison hemlock arrived in the United States and Canada comparatively recently. Now it grows as a weed that is quite easily mistaken for ordinary parsley and the root of wild carrot.

It is the seeds and the leaves that bear most of the deadly poison called conium, a pale volatile oily substance. Conium is a mixture of five deadly components, the most poisonous of which is one called coniine, which is also the one causing the symptoms of Socrates.

Foxglove

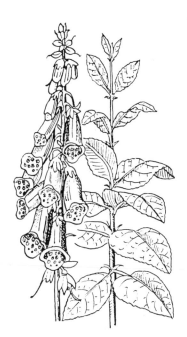

Foxglove (*Digitalis purpurea*).

The foxglove (*Digitalis purpurea*) is an attractive purple and white plant known around the world. From it came the original stores of the useful heart stimulant digitalis, which strengthens and slows down the heartbeat. Overdoses lead to nausea, distress in the stomach region, irregular heartbeat and eventually drowsiness and tremors. Decorative and useful it is, but it also has more than its fair share of legend and lore. In Ireland foxglove flowers are called "fairy caps." These are tiny caps worn by the Wee Folk as they cavort in the moonlight and dance to the tinkle of the "fairy bells," as they are shaken by the musical pixies. The Irish do not believe the foxglove plant bends under the weight of its flowers. Rather, it's the flower's way of making a curtsy to the Fairy Queen sitting nearby, invisible to mere mortals.

Jimson Weed

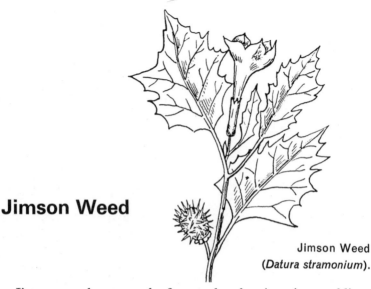

Jimson Weed
(*Datura stramonium*).

Jimson weed was made famous by the American soldiers in Jamestown who were sent to put down what historians call Bacon's Rebellion. This was in 1676 in the easternmost part of Colonial America. The soldiers, it seems, mistook the jimson weed for some edible plant and made it into a salad. The effects were remarkable. In a short while the whole army turned into a band of buffoons. Some blew feathers into the air, while others tried to shoot them down with straws, while still others sat around in their birthday suits grinning from ear to ear at the goings on. And so it was for 11 days (we are told), when things suddenly returned to normal and the whole incident was forgotten.

Considering what jimson weed has in it the Jamestown soldiers were very lucky. The constituent in jimson weed responsible for these actions is the delirium drug called "stramonine," actually made up of three separate compounds, namely hyoscyamine, atropine and scopolamine. Scopolamine at various times has been used as a truth serum and (reportedly) a brainwashing drug by some of the major powers.

110

Atropine is best known as the drug used by the doctor to widen the pupils of the eye.

An overdose of stramonium causes extreme thirst—thirst so great that no amount of water will satisfy it—enlarged pupils of the eye, excitement, delirium, jumbled speech and for all practical purposes a state of insanity. The insanity may be followed by convulsions and, in extreme overdoses, death.

Jimson weed (*Datura stramonium*) also goes by the names thornapple, devil's apple, stinkweed, stramonium and angel's trumpet. The name is a more popular version of "Jamestown weed."

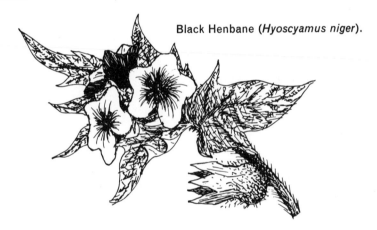

Black Henbane (*Hyoscyamus niger*).

Black Henbane

Black henbane has a reputation that goes back to ancient times but otherwise it has much in common with the jimson weed made famous in the time of Colonial America. The symptoms it produces are almost the same as the jimson weed, since they both contain the same components as in stramonine. There's a story that henbane was served by mistake in a medieval monastery in Europe one evening and that by midnight of that evening the bells were tolling, monks were walking about holding open books (which they couldn't possibly read), were singing bar-room songs and doing all the things the dignity of a monk would otherwise not allow.

Shakespeare called henbane "the cursed juice of Hebenon" in Hamlet, and Pliny, very much earlier, wrote that henbane "troubled the brain and bred dizziness in the head" and that it was "of the nature of wine, therefore offensive to the understanding."

These accusations are in no way out of line. Since ancient times this deadly flower was used to dull the sensations and to produce hallucinations. Toothache remedies, for instance, were made by boiling the root of henbane in vinegar and holding it in the mouth while still hot. Witches were able to conjure up visions and talk to the Spirits when they inhaled the smoke of tobacco and henbane. Then too they were prepared for the "Witches Sabbath" by an ointment made of henbane, mandragorium and belladonna. Rubbed over their bodies the ointment soon made them unconscious and when they woke up they believed they had visited Spiritland and had returned to Earth.

Mandragora

Mandragora is the poison (or medicine) from the root of the mandrake plant, a plant with beautiful purple flowers and a root that often resembles a human body.

In 1121 an Anglo-Saxon poet called Philip de Thaun wrote that the female root resembles a girl and that this plant had leaves like lettuce, and that the leaves of the plant with the male-shaped root had the regular leaves of the mandrake plant. He explained in great detail how the plant should be rooted from the ground and added that "when one has this root it is of great value in medicine, for it cures every infirmity—except death where there is no help. I will say no more about it. . . ."

People in the south of England firmly believed that the mandrake had a human heart in its root and that it was guarded

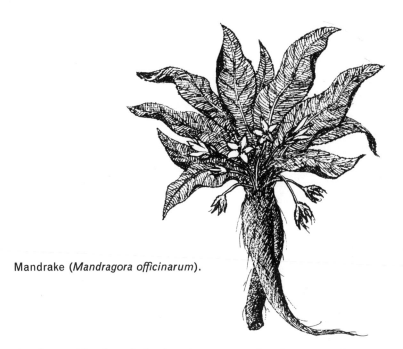

Mandrake (*Mandragora officinarum*).

by Satan. Further, it had to be uprooted only at certain holy days and then only according to the proper ritual. If this were done all would be well and Satan would do the plucker's bidding. Otherwise, the harvester would die within the year and he would die screaming, just as the mandrake plant did when he plucked it (another belief held that when the mandrake plant was uprooted it would shriek and moan like a human).

The mandrake was introduced into England from Europe during the reign of Henry VIII. Soon its roots were so valuable as love charms and witches' aids that the Briony root was substituted. There is a very strong resemblance.

The poison in the mandrake plant, called mandragorine, is a combination of the delirium drugs hyoscyamine and scopolamine, and acts much like the poisons in jimson weed, henbane and belladonna.

Mandragora was probably one of the first of the medical anesthetics. On the battlefields it was mixed with wine to dull the pain. This led to its use in civilian surgery later, according to Pliny. Prior to surgery, wrote Pliny, a dried anodyne of mandrake, opium, henbane, lettuce and camphor was reconstituted in steaming water. Then a loaded sponge was held to the nostrils of the victim until he slumbered.

Historical antidotes to mandrake poisoning include honey, radish, butter, oatmeal, rue, sweet wine, castoreum in old wine, borax, leaves of watermint, absinthe in old wine, asafetida, "and if that is not enough, add natron." The victim should have his head bound and rose oil poured into one nostril. Should this fail, pour mint and leaf of almond hot over his head while he sits in a bath. This may be followed by anointing him with a hot mixture of olive oil, water and sharp wine. Honeyed old raisin wine should be drunk during the latter treatment. Finally, a concoction of nutmeg, wild ginger, mastic, clove bark, nutmeg and cinnamon pulverized in hot wine to which is added saffron, nutmeg and black pepper, must be filtered and decanted as a water substitute where the victim is overtaken by terrible thirst. Such a remedy was costly.

Aconite: Queen Mother of Poisons

To the ancients aconite was Queen Mother of poisons. It was their most poisonous and important plant. In the two thousand years of its acquaintance with man it has gone under various names, including wolfsbane, leopard's bane, women's bane, devil's helmet and monkshood. The rural English called it "the flower with the pretty blue bonnet" and in North America it is the garden flower with a bonnet like the hood of a monastery monk, that is, a "monkshood." Its scientific name is *Aconitum napellus* and the name "aconite" is

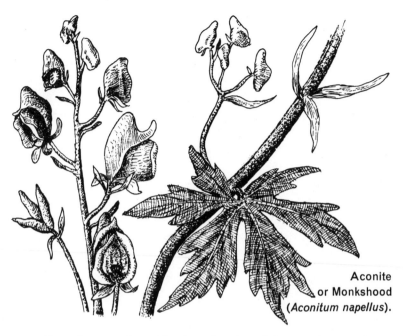

Aconite
or Monkshood
(*Aconitum napellus*).

attributed to ancient Greeks who found it growing on bare rocks, which they called "aconas."

Call it what we will, we won't change its devilish nature. In olden times it was described by one writer as a root which "doth turn and crook inward in the manner of a scorpions taile." Above ground monkshood is often mistaken for watercress. Recently a 23-year-old man on a nature walk with a companion in the dense woods some miles north of Santa Cruz, California, ate two monkshood plants, thinking they were watercress. According to his companion he was dead at the scene within 15 minutes.

Monkshood produces tingling of the mouth, throat and face when first chewed. Larger amounts would also produce a cold clammy skin, numbness of the mouth and throat, giddiness, slow heart action, loss of muscular power and a strange sense of doom experienced just before death. This all happens between eight minutes and three or four hours after eating.

The total amount of aconite need not be more than 1 milligram.

The name of the deadly compound is aconitine. Its final effect is to cause the muscles which control breathing to become paralyzed.

How Aconite Came To Be: A Mythological Beginning

Medea the Sorceress and Poisoner became the wife of the King of Athens. Theseus the son of Aegeus was raised outside the kingdom but it was preordained that he return at the rightful time and claim his honors and someday the throne. Moreover Theseus was to be recognized by the sword given him by Aegeus when he was born—the King's own sword. As the time approached Theseus wanted to learn if he would really be welcomed so he went ahead in disguise. Medea however learned of his coming and, as she feared Theseus would interfere with her control of the kingdom, she told the King that the stranger was really a spy and came to do only harm. "When you hand the stranger the welcome goblet," she said, "it must have poison in it."

The King agreed; whereupon Medea went to her poison garden but couldn't find a herb strong enough. So she stamped her foot and caused aconite to spring forth. She then put the juice of the aconite plant into the goblet of wine and handed it to the King as the stranger came forward to be welcomed at the throne. But just as the stranger reached for the goblet his sword fell to the marble floor and the King having recognized it instantly knew that Theseus was really his son. He threw the goblet to the marble floor in great anger. As the tale ends the wine soaked into the marble and aconite plants sprang forth from the site and Medea fled in great haste on a chariot drawn by her dragons.

The ancient physician Malthiolus was commissioned by Pope Clement VII to develop an antidote for, according to the Pope, "the most deadly poison known." Malthiolus was offered criminals condemned to die to develop his antidote for aconite. To two groups he gave a poison and to only one of the groups the antidote of the moment. No statistics were needed to determine the effect (if any). His antidotes were many and complicated but the one which seemed to work best was a mixture of oil and water. We know that this usually causes the victim to throw up and remove most of the poison not yet absorbed—which is probably the antidote's only claim to success.

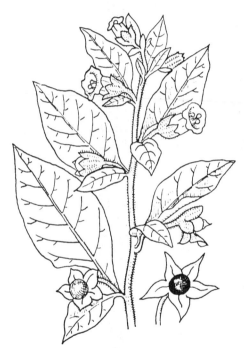

Belladonna

Belladonna (*Atropa belladonna*).

Another deadly flower, belladonna, is also known by other names: poison cherry, naughty man's cherries, devil's herb and sorcerer's herb. Translated from the Italian it means "beautiful woman," for it has long been intimately associated with feminine beauty.

Medieval and ancient ladies put a drop of belladonna juice in each eye to enlarge the pupil. They understood already what modern psychologists have recently demonstrated in the cold atmosphere of the laboratory. A series of photographs were shown to a group of men. Each showed a beautiful woman identical in every way with the others except that the pupils in the eyes of one woman were very large. Invariably this picture was selected as that of the most beautiful woman. Poker players know the meaning of large pupils. They look into the eyes of their opponents, for, without fail, the sight of a "good hand" widens the pupil and, for the same reason, *they* may wear dark glasses. Chinese jade dealers and commodity sharpies do much the same. They know that when a prospective customer's pupils widen he likes the merchandise, whereupon the price goes up.

Belladonna (*Atropa belladonna*) has a long and shady history. The ancient Greeks believed it to be the chosen plant of Circe the Sorceress, and people of medieval Europe believed that Satan guarded it at all times—except on very special occasions. It differed with countries but in Germany it was *Walpurgisnacht* (April 30) and on a certain night when Satan was drawn off guard by a black hen which he couldn't resist chasing. It was only then that the plant could be picked in safety. Belladonna too was one of the main ingredients in the witches "Flying Ointment," used to propel the well known broomstick aloft.

Castor Bean

One of Hawaii's many ornamental plants is the castor bean (*Ricinus communis*). At times it grows into a large tree, the seeds of which are processed for the castor oil they contain. But in the raw, unprocessed condition the seeds of this tree contain a powerful poison called ricin. The seeds themselves could be swallowed whole with no effect, *but* if as little as 1/100

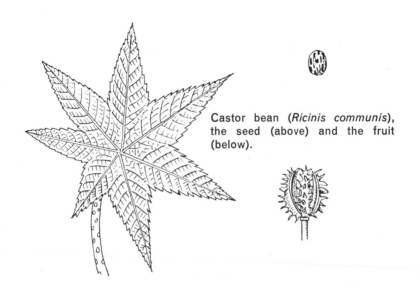

Castor bean (*Ricinis communis*), the seed (above) and the fruit (below).

of a milligram gets into the blood it becomes a fatal dose. Ricin clumps together red blood cells and causes bleeding on the inside as well as severe kidney damage and other dangerous effects.

Rosary Peas

Rosary peas (*Abrus precatorius*) are also called rosary beans, jequirity, love beads and precatory beans. They hang on vines and grow in pods like ordinary garden peas, but there the resemblance ends. Rosary peas are used only for jewelry, beads, necklaces and bracelets. Being about $\frac{1}{4}$ inch (6 millimetres) long and brightly colored—orange at one end and jet black on the other—they make attractive and safe jewelry *unless* the wearer perspires. Then the natural perspiration may cause some of the poisonous compound called abrin to be absorbed through the skin. Ordinarily the beans have a hard coating and could be swallowed with no ill effects but if only *one* bean is chewed and swallowed death is almost certain. Abrin of the rosary peas and ricin of the castor beans are similar in their effects. Symptoms may not develop immediately on swallowing or may not even appear for several days but following this lapse of time there's a loss of appetite, stomach upset, delirium and finally total collapse. There is no known antidote.

Fields of Poppies

What could be more peaceful and tranquil than a distant mountain-side with its fields of poppies swaying gently in the summer breeze? Everything about the poppy suggests the peace of an unreal world. Greek mythology associated the poppy with Nyx (the goddess of night), Hypnos (the god of sleep), Thanatos (the god of death) and Morpheus (the god of dreams). And the scientific name too suggests sleep: Somnus, the Roman god of sleep, clearly forms a part of *Papaver somniferum.*

A worldwide desire to escape suffering and the harsh demands of existence is anything but new. In the Ebers Papyrus, one of the earliest known records of medicine, there is mention of the opium of the poppy plant. The papyrus dates back to 1550 B.C. Egyptians of this era preferred it with wine, hot pepper and other aromatic spices. When they were denied what they called their "Cretic Wine" they suffered a condition they called faintness and languidness.

Sometime during the ninth century the Arabs introduced opium to India and several other countries. Later one of its greatest cities, Bengal, became the world's center for opium production. Greedy Indian merchants wanted to dispose of the burgeoning supplies so the East India Company sponsored oriental "bootleggers," British agents and an assortment of gangsters and pushers to stir up China—a huge prospective market for the Indian opium. But the Chinese government didn't take kindly to this interference and the Opium War of

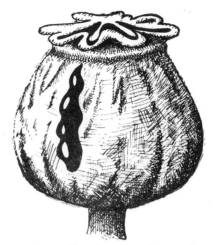

When properly tapped, the poppy yields a stream of yellowish-brown opium.

1839 was on. It lasted three years, ending in easy victory for the British. Soon the number of Chinese opium eaters began to increase and a hundred years later a fifth of China was active in eating or smoking opium.

Opium is the juice of the white poppy as taken from the head of a poppy. (Nonwhite varieties yield opium too, but not nearly as much.) The dried rubbery material on the head contains about twenty different compounds. The most abundant and potent of these compounds is morphine (approximately 10 per cent of the total).

In Southeast Asia entire fields of white and purple poppies are tapped between the months of December and February. A few days after the petals fall, the capsule—a greenish, squashed bulb—is carefully examined by the native specialist. Scarring a poppy is also a most exacting art. A small curved blade is used by the native experts to make an incision. If the incision is too deep fluid runs to the ground; if not deep enough it will harden in the capsule. Moreover this must all take place under a bright sun. When properly scarred a yellowish-brown mass results. This is scraped off and collected on rice paper or a banana leaf and stored for future destinations.

The West was as inclined toward escapism as the Orient. But in the West it was not opium but rather its active components which took hold.

It all started rather innocently. Morphine, an extract of opium, was used by physicians to kill pain. The famous physician, William Osler, even referred to morphine as "God's own medicine" when speaking of its pain-killing powers. Doctors began to depend on it medically, and patients physically and mentally. Then in 1848 a new technical invention

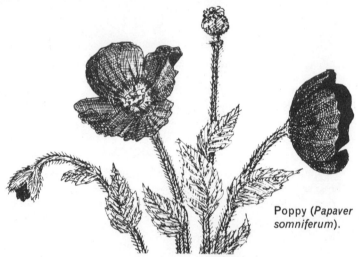

Poppy (*Papaver somniferum*).

seemed to provide a safe method for physicians to prescribe morphine. It was thought that the needle would stop addiction because it was no longer necessary for morphine to go through the stomach. Unfortunately when morphine is injected directly and the stomach bypassed the effect is twenty-two times as powerful. Then too it was almost on a do-it-yourself basis. No longer was there a need to buy prepared medicine— everything was available at the corner drug store. In 1874 a German doctor by the name of Heinrich Dreser discovered what he thought was a "cure" for morphine addiction. He called this "cure" heroin, after the Greek god Heros and he

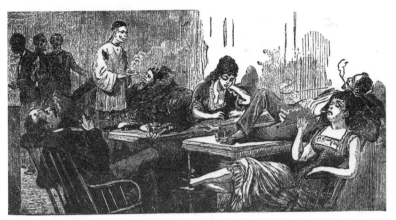

The Western world enthusiastically accepted narcotics, as in this scene from an aristocratic opium den.

though it would benefit all mankind. For this reason heroin was more than enthusiastically prescribed for addiction to opium and morphine. This turned out to be one of the colossal mistakes of history, for in a few months it was realized that not only does heroin cause addiction but that it is two and a half times as strong as morphine. In 1898 it was estimated that there were 1.4 million Americans on some form of opium. The problem of drug abuse throughout the world since the turn of the century has been a gigantic one.

The Oleander Tree

The oleander (*Nerium oleander*) is a shrub-like tree that bears beautiful pink or white blossoms throughout much of the year and grows to a height of some 20 feet (6 metres). It's abundant throughout the South and West of the United States and in Canada, being used as decorative hedges on estates, in yards and along highways.

The poison contained in the oleander tree is a heart stimulant (like digitalis) so powerful that a single leaf well chewed is fatal to man. The poison called oleanderside is contained in all parts of the plant. There was a beach party of a dozen or so persons which ended in tragedy. Oleander twigs were used as spits to roast hot dogs in the open fire. Poison evidently distilled out of the twigs into the hot dogs, for the whole group was found dead at the scene. Numerous such incidents were reported in military records, where soldiers in the field use what seems to be most convenient.

Symptoms are similar to those of a digitalis overdose; that is, nausea, drowsiness, slow pulse, irregular heart beat, unconsciousness and finally paralysis of the muscles that control breathing.

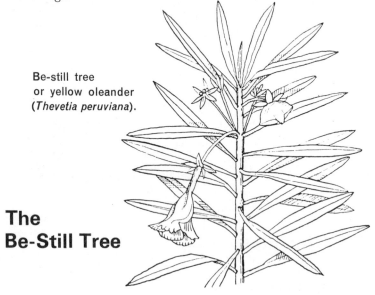

Be-still tree
or yellow oleander
(*Thevetia peruviana*).

The
Be-Still Tree

The be-still tree is an ornamental tree with bright yellow and orange flowers at the branch tips. It is called the be-still tree because the leaves seem to quiver in place when even the slightest breeze stirs them. Though attractive, the tree is also a major cause of poisoning in the Hawaiian paradise of Oahu. All parts of it contain the deadly poison thevetin, which acts much like the heart stimulant digitalis.

124

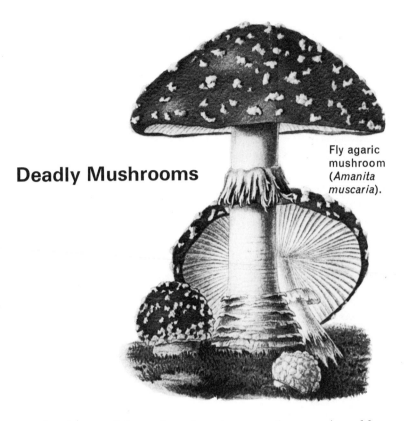

Deadly Mushrooms

Fly agaric mushroom (*Amanita muscaria*).

There's something miraculous in a mushroom. A sudden spring shower and a whole field of mushrooms appear where the evening before there was not one. Such a ghostly manifestation is hard to understand. The ancients explained it by saying the mushrooms sprang from a bolt of night lightning. Mushrooms are considered miraculous by some because they seem to push secret buttons in the mind and reveal scenes directly from another world. The trips to paradise can be one way trips, though, for only mushrooms of the deadliest clans have this power.

One of the deadly types is the fly agaric (*Amanita muscaria*). The fly agaric got its name from the fact that it contains a substance irresistible to flies. It is sought after for the hallucinogenic poison called muscarine. In small amounts it is used by people the world over to create visions and the atmosphere needed for various rituals and ceremonies. In amounts of about 120 milligrams or over (for an adult) it can remove a person completely—and permanently. Muscarine is a fast-acting poison that can cause the nervous system to be overstimulated. Symptoms appear almost immediately after eating: sweating, wheezing, irregular breathing and heart action and mental confusion. It turns out that the poison acts so fast that it causes vomiting almost immediately, eliminating most of the poison before it can be absorbed to a significant extent.

The deadliest mushroom in the world is the death cup (*Amanita phalloides*). It is also known by the names destroying angel and spring amanita. Once its poison enters the bloodstream there's nothing that can be done. True, several cases of survival have been reported but, as in the case of rabies, the odds are none too good. The reason is that the death cup contains, actually, five poisons. One is called phalloidin. It takes 50 millionths of a gram to kill a full grown laboratory mouse and is four times as potent as cyanide. It is a slow poison which produces a sudden seizure of abdominal pain about 12 hours or so after eating. If the victim is lucky enough to survive this ordeal he will feel much better for some six to eight days. Then the other poisons, one of which is called alpha-amanitine, start grinding away at any last hope. Amanitine is far more powerful than the phalloidin, requiring only 2 millionths of a gram to remove the laboratory mouse, about 25 thousandths the weight of a drop of water and a hundred times as strong as cyanide. Amanitine and the other less potent poisons then start to shut the kidney down and begin to disintegrate the liver cells. Later the mind hallucinates and finally the brain dies. It is an ordeal that is beyond adequate description.

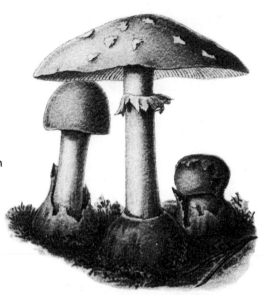

Death cup mushroom
(*Amanita phalloides*).

A variety of claims have been made for an antidote to the death cup but there has so far always been a dispute over the reliability of the data presented. As understanding increases, however, so do the chances of success. In the meantime the thing to do is to avoid the problem in the first place!

The Strychnine Tree

Several tall trees growing in Hawaii go by the name of *Strychnos nux vomica*. This is the tree which produced the first strychnine. Two especially attractive ones grow in a park at Keeaumoku and King Streets and in the Foster Gardens of Nuuanu. These trees bear a fruit that looks like a velvet-covered button. The poisonous strychnine can be found in any part of the tree, blossoms and all, but the highest concentration is in the buttons. Blossoms, however, smell like curry and are at times a somewhat dangerous though attractive nuisance to children.

Exotic Poisons of Nature: Deadly Minerals and Chemical Creations

> Time poisons work slowly but wipe out their victims just
> the same. Even worse, the victim isn't aware that he's being
> poisoned until the very last moments. In this sense slow
> poisons may be as strangely different and fascinating—
> exotic—as their fast-acting counterparts. And like most
> other poisons they are at once remedies and tools for evil,
> substances of the world and the occult. Famous and
> representative mineral poisons and simple but important
> compounds follow, among them the possibly perfect
> poisoner's poison.

Arsenic, the Preferred Poison

Arsenic was known to the ancient Egyptians, Assyrians,
Hebrews and Greeks since sometime before the fifth century
B.C., but it experienced its peak of popularity in the Middle
Ages. Pope Clement VII (in 1534) was poisoned by fumes as
he carried a candle in a religious procession. Arsenic was
blended into the wax of the candle (and probably changed into
a more volatile form by the heat and the hydrogen gas coming
off with it). In 1705 Leopold I of Austria was also removed by
the fumes of an arsenic-laden candle.

More popular methods were to mix arsenic with food and
drink. Some one or two hours after taking on a fatal dose the
victim experienced what seemed to be symptoms of the stomach
flu. In the Middle Ages and before it gave the same symptoms
as the widespread disease called cholera, which was much like
the flu except that the symptoms were more exaggerated and

were usually fatal. Being so, no questions were asked and death was attributed to cholera. Seasoning food and drink this way is possible because arsenic is odorless and tasteless and is fairly heavy, so that the dose amounts to only a small pinch. (There are 7 grains (450 milligrams) to the teaspoonful. This would be roughly 4 times the fatal dose.) Arsenic poisoners often preferred to give doses as a series of larger and larger amounts or as the same amount spaced at closer intervals. This was to throw off suspicion, get the victim used to the slight aftertaste and to begin tearing down the foundation of his ability to resist the final overdose, which was given at some opportune time chosen by the poisoner.

Is it possible to build up a tolerance for arsenic by taking increasingly larger doses over a long interval of time? It seems so. The Aztecs claim to have immunity (but only up to a point). As children they begin to eat arsenic regularly. It is said that their unusual skin color is caused by the peculiar interaction between the sun and the arsenic under their skins. And there are peasants in Styria who are supposed to eat arsenic just for the fun of it. It improves their complexions, gives them sleek hair and improves their wind (or so they claim). It is known that some peasants can put away doses lethal several times over for an ordinary person. It appears likely that such a tolerance could be developed over a long period—say a year or so— but it is well to remember that tribal knowledge of dosages and methods was accumulated over a long history involving trial and error and many non-successes. Moreover, the form of arsenic is important to consider: the powder form used by the natives is not as harmful as the kidney-damaging liquid forms.

Hippocrates (460–377 B.C.), the father of medicine, used arsenic to cure a number of illnesses. The form he used was the yellow form, which smells a lot like garlic. This would hardly suit the requirements of the secretive poisoner. What we usually mean by the word "arsenic" is the white form (also called arsenious oxide) which is both tasteless and odorless (if pure enough). It was in the 8th century that the Arabian alchemist Jabir iben Hayyan first distilled the white form from the yellow form and launched the most popular poison on its way.

Quicksilver

Mercury had been known in Egypt since before 1550 B.C. and probably even earlier in India and China. Around the fourth century B.C. in Greece, Aristotle called mercury "Quicksilver," for that's what it seemed like to the eye. But the ancient alchemists were the first to call mercury "Mercury," after the most wily and fleetfooted of the Roman gods. Mercury was known for its occult powers in 17th and 18th century England, where it was common practice to carry a vial of mercury to guard against rheumatism. A writer by the name of Woodal, in 1639, briefly captured Nature's only liquid element in words. He wrote: "It is the hottest, the coldest, a true healer, a wicked murderer, a precious medicine and a deadly poison. . . ." Yet mercury is more. It appears throughout nature, in rocks, soil, air and water.

Why does mercury appear almost everywhere? Probably because it was formed billions of years ago along with the other elements and has worked its way to the surface in the form of veins of pure "quicksilver" or as such natural compounds as cinnabar (the sulfide of mercury, its most common form). Land erosion washed it into the oceans which today contain some 50 million tons (45 million tonnes) of the metal. But changes are not likely to be detected easily. Tests show that the mercury level of the oceans is the same now as it was a hundred years ago (and it would be safe to say a thousand or ten thousand). In the sea fishes and mammals convert some of the mineral forms into organic forms (compounds with the element carbon somewhere in their makeup). Moreover, micro-organisms in the mud of the ocean or river floors assist in the change of form.

In some rivers and bodies of water on the receiving end of certain industrial waste products the level of mercury may be much higher, for mercury is more widely used than it may seem at first glance. Consider just a few instances: the making of thermometers, fluorescent light bulbs, energy cells for wrist watches, farm products like fertilizers, fungicides and disinfectants, medicines and cosmetics and such industrial processes as the preparation of chlorine for swimming pools, and so on. These thousands upon thousands of tons find their way into water, earth or junkyards.

There are two kinds of mercury poisoning. The first and less serious is caused by the mineral forms, usually brought on by breathing the vapor of metallic mercury. Irritation of the mouth and throat areas and damage to the cells of the kidney usually result. The second is caused by an organic form called methyl mercury, as is occasionally found in sea foods. Brain damage and damage to the central nervous system and the chromosomes result. It's necessary to absorb about one milligram of mercury daily for some two or three months before any symptoms show up. These are numbness, considerable crankiness, forgetfulness and damage to the brain and other organs which eventually bring about unconsciousness and death. The sinister feature in mercury poisoning is that the onset is so slow that the victims simply feel bad but (as most will say) they "don't know what's wrong."

Common Carbon Monoxide

Carbon monoxide is a simple compound consisting of one atom of carbon and one of oxygen (CO). *Any* amount is dangerous in the sense that it immobilizes some red blood cells, but there's no way to avoid it completely, for the average concentration in the world's atmosphere varies between 0.1 and 1.0 parts per million (ppm). Most of this is contributed by nature through the decay of plants and evaporation from the oceans. This amounts to 3.5 billion tons (3.15 billion tonnes) in one year and in the northern hemisphere alone. This is 12 or 13 times as much as that which comes from automobile exhausts and other man-made sources: that is, 270 million tons (245 million tonnes) each year.

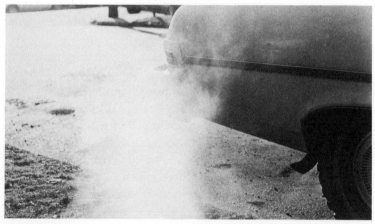

In areas of heavy automobile traffic, the level of carbon monoxide in the air often reaches dangerous levels for several hours at a time.

Each car produces on the average 3,200 pounds (1,400 kilograms) a year. No wonder cities like Tokyo and Los Angeles have concentrations some 50 times the average level in air far removed from automobile exhaust. City streets often have 30 parts per million for hours at a time and often peak out at a hundred ppm. American Federal Air Standards limit continuous exposure to air with 9 ppm to an eight hour period, for at this level 2% of the blood's red cells are immobilized and symptoms of poisoning appear—headaches, for example. A four hour exposure at 100 ppm immobilizes 12% of the red cells; at 300 ppm, 35% and at 750 ppm 60%. This exposure would destroy brain cells by withholding oxygen (just as in drowning) and results in permanent damage.

Half of the 12,000 yearly deaths of fire victims in the U.S. are attributed to carbon monoxide but in a rather indirect way. Poisonous fumes and gases from burning plastics and other materials cause carbon monoxide poisoning by confusing the fire victims as they try to escape. A fire involving plastics (among other things) will cause the liberation of toxic fumes, among them hydrogen cyanide, phosgene (the World War I gas), nitrogen oxides, chlorine and many other less dangerous gases.

Lead

Hippocrates, the physician of ancient Greece, described illnesses of workers in the smelting industries, alchemists through the ages were aware of lead poisoning and in 1700 a medical writer named Romazzini referred to lead poisoning in a book called *Diseases of Tradesmen*. True, lead poisoning has been known since biblical times, but in a sense it's a modern problem and one especially likely to affect children. In America 400,000 children have higher levels of lead in their blood than they should have. Of this number 32,000 will suffer some sort of brain damage, 800 will be permanently damaged and 200 will die. A likely place for children to get lead is from paint chips or flakes. A 1974 law requires that paints have less than 0.06% lead, but this lead-free paint may merely cover several layers of older paint. It takes only a fingernail-size chip of paint nibbled at frequently over a period of months to exceed the allowable level of lead in the blood (set to be less than a total average daily intake of 300 micrograms from all sources). A study of 6,000 children in the Chicago area revealed 18.6% had high lead levels. Another likely source for children is the lead in the cans used for milk. One particular study showed 200 micrograms of lead in one can or two thirds of the maximum allowed for 1 to 3 year olds (300 micrograms). Then too, it has been found that the concentration of lead is twice as high in the first 4 feet (1.2 metres) of air above ground as it is from there on up. Children, of course, would then breathe in air with a higher lead content than adults. Lead from gasoline, however, is a source of lead that plagues adults, for it contaminates vegetation, house dust, clothes and anything bathed in the leaded air. Pencils and pottery are two other sources of lead. A new regulation to reduce the lead content of pencils to less than 0.5% in the U.S. has been passed but no regulation on pottery imported from Mexico and other countries is workable. A California family, for instance, was poisoned by orange juice served out of earthenware pottery. It seems that the acid of the juice leached out the lead. (Fully glazed pottery is strongly recommended by health authorities.)

Lead poisoning is the kind that builds up gradually. Lead

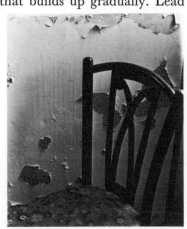

A prime source
of lead poisoning in children
is peeling lead-base paint.

can be dissolved in the body fluids and stored in the body indefinitely. It is dangerous *only* when it is in circulation or when it leaves the body cells in which it is stored. Symptoms of lead poisoning include headache, irritability, loss of red blood cells, a feeling of sluggishness and in more severe exposures brain damage, blindness, kidney damage, convulsions and death.

One of the bright spots of late is a test so sensitive that one drop of blood, a marvelously responsive chemical and a fluorescent light bulb will detect 5 trillionths (5 ppt) of a gram of lead.

Ancient Antimony

Use of antimony has faded from visible use into various disguises, in the compositions of countless industrial alloys and compounds. But in the workshops of the 16th and 17th centuries, it was made into "antimony cups." These were vessels of antimony in which wine was allowed to stand for days or weeks. The "tartar of wine" became the "tartar of antimony," a substance known to cause a victim to throw up. (There's the story that monastery monks were often guilty of over-indulging in wine, and as punishment they were required to drink one more from "the cup," whereupon they would become ill enough to throw up and repent.) Overdoses of antimony lead to death, not illness. Antimony was also used to remove condemned criminals.

Cyanide and Two Perfect Crimes

Cyanide is found in many of nature's products. Leaves of the wild black cherry tree (*Prunus secrotina*) contain a substance called amygdalin which, when broken down by the enzymes of the stomach, yields hydrogen cyanide in great enough quantity so that only several leaves (well chewed) can cause death "within the hour." It is well known that seeds of apples, peaches, plums, apricots, cherries, and almonds are high in cyanide-laden compounds. There's the story of a man who loved apple seeds so much that he saved them religiously. When he had one cupful he ate them all at once—and died within minutes of his apple seed orgy.

Cyanide is a simple chemical compound of one atom of carbon joined to one atom of nitrogen. These must be joined to another atom such as hydrogen. In this form (HCN) it is called prussic acid, or hydrogen cyanide gas, an invisible form (supposedly) with the smell of bitter almonds. It acts directly on the nervous system, and very rapidly. Its action is based on stopping the use of oxygen by the tissue cells and its paralysis of the center of the brain which controls the breathing muscles. Its maximum allowable concentration is only 5 ppm in air. Prison gas chambers were operated by dropping cyanide eggs (pellets of sodium cyanide) into a vessel of water and sulfuric acid. The reaction liberated prussic acid and with a few convulsive movements it was "all over."

Cyanide has been used to commit the perfect crime by Leonardo da Vinci, among others. Leonardo was most famous as a 15th century painter but he was also an all-around genius who put a touch of originality on everything he did. That this applied to perfectionism in poisoning and the work of the sorcerer is not too well known. A biography by the Russian writer Merezhkovski related Leonardo's perfect crime.

The great painter, according to Merezhkovski, was such a skilled poisoner that he anticipated a technique which later became known as the "passages." Four steps were involved in the method of passages:

- Killing an animal by injecting a poison.
- Removing the organs impregnated—usually the heart, spleen or lungs.
- Preparing an extract using these organs.
- Introducing the poisonous extract into another animal.

With each passage the strength of the poison increased. What Leonardo did was to apply this method to plants. He injected the potassium form of cyanide (KCN in chemical symbols) under the bark of fruit trees in increasingly larger doses. The fruit—apples, pears, peaches or cherries—contained small quantities of cyanide, small enough not to cause death. It had to be eaten for weeks before it would be fatal.

Fruit from Leonardo's garden was served at a banquet in

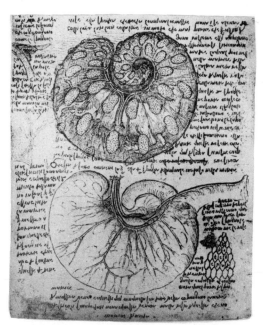

Leonardo's drawings of human organs demonstrate the biological knowledge which made him an expert poisoner.

the house of Lodovico il Moro to a Giangaleazzo Sforza. Sforza was sent more fruit for several days after the banquet, until—finally—he "yielded his soul to God."

THE PERFECT POISON?

What then makes an ideal poison for criminal purposes? Criminologists pretty well agree that the poison should:

- vanish from the victim before it can be detected by chemical analysis (This consideration depends on *when* the poisoning was done. In olden times no scientific tests were possible and often suspicion was not even aroused, for one reason or another.)
- have no antidote
- be tasteless and odorless
- be effective in minuscule amounts
- have a delayed reaction—delayed enough to give the poisoner a chance to cover his tracks.

137

> Situations and preferences vary, but it may be that the perfect poison is a substance considered not to be poisonous at all—the gas given off by the kind of dry ice familiar to summer picnickers. The gas is called carbon dioxide. Consider this crime: A block of dry ice is placed above the sleeping victim in such a way that the heavy vapors flow down and displace the air surrounding the victim. This would deprive him of any oxygen and cause him to suffocate in his sleep.

Years ago a Russian spy committed the "perfect crime" using cyanide and its antidote. His perfect crime was revealed in *Famous Soviet Spies*, a recent account by Joseph Newman.

On October 9, 1957 a slight young man with a thin face and light blue eyes checked into the Stachus Hotel in Munich, Germany. He seemed to be an unobtrusive guest in a modest hotel. On the register he appeared as Siegfried Kruger but his real name was Bogdon Stashynasky and inside his coat pocket was a strange weapon. He had a contract to kill. Like himself, his intended victim, a Lev Rebet, was from the Ukraine. Five years before, Rebet's execution had been contracted for at a Soviet Security staff meeting. Rebet, a heavy-set, energetic middle-aged man was a popular Ukranian exiled political leader and editor of an anti-Soviet newspaper, the *Ukrainski Samastinik*. He was described to Stashynasky as a "very dangerous man." Stashynasky had been to Munich twice before, in April and July of that year, to watch Rebet's movements. He had been equipped by a Moscow technical expert with a weapon he had not seen before. The weapon was a seven-inch metal tube that could be broken down into three sections. The first section held a firing pin, powered by a $1\frac{1}{2}$-volt battery, which made its action completely noiseless. Instead of bullets it fired the contents of a pellet containing the deadly prussic acid compound called potassium cyanide. The poison was completely invisible and odorless. Anyone who breathed it would be dead in seconds and long before an autopsy could be performed all traces of it would vanish. "It has been used with 100% success," the Moscow technical expert informed Stashynasky. "For your safety and protection you swallow one of these sodium thiosulphate tablets before shooting the gun," he added, "and then, immediately after firing, you crush this amyl nitrate ampoule and inhale." [The compound should be amyl nitrite rather than amyl nitrate . . . probably a misprint in the report.]

Stashynasky had an unpleasant duty to perform. He took up an inconspicuous position near a trolley stop and waited for Rebet's arrival. Each morning for three days he breakfasted on the antidote pill, took the spray gun from its container, wrapped it in a piece of newspaper, put it inside his coat pocket, and waited. On the third day assassin met victim. They both walked to the same building. Stashynasky reached the building before Rebet. He entered and went up the rickety stairs to the first floor. In the silent, dimly lit corridor he stood and waited, breathing hard. The sound of the front door opening came to him as a thunderous echo. He took the gun out of his pocket, unscrewed the safety lock, and started down the stairs. The older man climbed up the staircase, the victim to the assassin. As they met, Rebet's eyes shone—with just a faintly quizzical gleam. Stashynasky's right hand moved. He pointed, fired. There was a deadly hiss. Rebet gasped and fell forward. His murderer raced down the steps, paused long enough to crush his amyl nitrate pellet and inhale its contents, and walked casually along the street. Much later he circled back and noticed a crowd gathered in front of the building and a police car near the entrance. Lev Rebet was found dead on the stairs of his apartment, and the victim, according to records, died of "heart failure."*

*From *Famous Soviet Spies*, © 1973, U.S. News & World Report, Inc., Washington, D.C. 20037.

Protecting the Public from Poisons

> Governments around the world are attempting through regulation and research to cut down the tremendous number of deaths by poisoning. The development of safer packaging of commercial products has helped prevent the poisonings from happening. Once a poison has been taken, the modern network of poison control centers provides the information which often makes the difference between life and death.

Read the Label!

One of the most basic ways to protect against accidental poisoning—and one of the most frequently ignored—is to read the label of the products you use. The information on the label will warn of possible safety hazards and, in the event of accidental poisoning, will provide instant identification of the poison involved to the hospital, doctor or poison control center.

Labels contain several important items of information. They tell what the brand is: DRANO liquid drain opener, EARTHEWARE beauty shampoo, and so on. This is necessary information for the poison control center. They match this name with the composition on file in the computer and base their recommended action on the facts. Labels contain other pieces of information, depending on the type of product.

Items like shampoo will contain little information other than the brand name and the fact that it is a shampoo (advertising doesn't count). However, dangerous substances like drain openers must post warnings, list contents and indicate emergency action.

Over-the-counter drugs indicate brand name, the manufacturer, his address, the ingredient(s), dose, recommended use, cautions and warnings. Prescription drugs give the name of the pharmacy, its address and phone number, the doctor, prescription number, name of drug, to whom issued and the dose recommended.

Even when information is present it is often conveniently ignored. A label reads, for instance: "Don't use (poison X) for any purpose other than specified on this label." This means that testing has been strictly limited and using it for any other purpose is another way of playing "Russian roulette." A farmer ignored instructions on a label which said something to the effect that the insecticide he was about to use was not cleared for spraying in pastures. He lost a quarter of his herd of cattle.

In another case a farmer ignored what a label did say. The label recommended a certain dosage of insecticide for delousing cattle. The insecticide was a spray type. The farmer ignored what the label said and used several times the recommended dosage. At the same time he did something that the label didn't say to do. He sprayed his cattle in a closed shed, a technique farmers call "fogging." As the insecticide was not intended for fogging it was improperly used. His double barrel mistake cost him several calves.

Another farmer committed the cardinal sin. He used the material of an *unlabelled* container bought at an auction a year earlier. (This is playing Russian roulette with *all* the chambers loaded.) As it turned out the material in the bottle was parathion, undoubtedly the most deadly pesticide ever concocted by man (two drops absorbed through the skin causes death in man). The sad fact is that this particular farmer lost his entire herd.

Manufacturers of poisons sometimes clearly label their products as the poisons they are, as the law requires, but often they are merely going through the motions. Many garden insecticides, for instance, have labels with instructions in small print or obscure language. Sometimes the label is easily soiled, or it falls off, or it is "eaten" off by the noxious ingredients. At other times products are put into bottles that make them look more like groceries than insecticides. It is a fact that most prescription drugs are not nearly as dangerous as garden insecticides, yet prescription drugs are well labelled while insecticides and other common household poisons are not.

MR. YUK AND THE WORDLESS LABEL

Question: How can we label products for children who won't or can't read?

The Mr. Yuk label is the most effective safety measure yet devised for small children (this means the label and the parent's "no-no" instructions). The biggest reason for its effectiveness is that it was designed by children and for children, with a good steering committee of mothers and teachers. The objective was to find an image that a child under 5 years old could easily identify with and could instantly recognize as a "no-no."

Mr. Yuk was designed to show children that poison is "yukky."

The old skull and crossbones was rejected because it has lost its meaning, for it appears on T-shirts, pirate flags and any number of other items. To get to the heart of the matter young children were asked what they thought of when they heard the word "poison." They replied that poison can kill, it makes you sick, and mothers yell if you play with it. Researchers realized that children are hard to scare—they delight in horror movies. They seem to be unshakable. But the tests showed that there was one sensation that repulsed them all—throwing up. *This* is what the picture of Mr. Yuk reminds them of. This and the ghastly green color made the perfect "turn off" signal. (The name, incidentally, is said to have come from a little boy who said it looked "Yukky.")

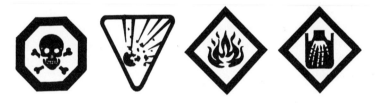

These symbols, in use in Canada, combine pictures representing different types of dangerous substances with different shapes indicating the degree of danger..

Canada's Department of Consumer and Corporate Affairs favors pictorial warnings on hazardous products of all types. The Department provides a leaflet explaining the meaning of the four symbols used to warn people about hazardous products, along with detachable symbols to be pasted on home supplies of drain cleaner, cleaning fluid, furniture polish, gasoline, drugs, medicines and so on. The skull and crossbones warns against poisons; an exploding bomb against the possibilities of an explosion; leaping flames against fires; and the skeleton of a hand against highly corrosive fluid. These four symbols are combined with three basic shapes: the octagon—meaning "real danger if the product is misused"; the diamond—meaning "warning"; and the triangle—meaning "take caution."

PROTECTOR TOPS

Protector tops are a recent innovation in the child safety area. The American Society for Testing Materials was responsible for developing various ingenious methods for protecting children from poisons in bottles. These methods were to follow the results of the Food and Drug Administration's Child Panel Test for Safety Enclosures. The "panel" involved some 200 children between 42 and 51 months. A closure was considered safe if 85% of the children were unable to open it within 5 minutes without instruction. With instruction 80% of the children had to be unable to open it within 5 minutes.

Safety closures are not always popular with adults. They're bothersome. If no small children are around, caps are often left off or in a loose position. Moreover, people with disabilities, such as arthritis, can't open and close the lids.

"Universal Antidote Kits"

Universal antidote kits are available at most drugstores or pharmaceutical counters in other stores. They come under names such as UNIDOTE and REACT. Most contain an ounce of activated charcoal and very simple instructions for its use in emergencies. Physicians recommend 1–2 tablespoons (15–30 millilitres) of activated charcoal in a glass of water, usually after the stomach has been emptied by vomiting, which is induced by an emetic, like syrup of ipecac.

HOMEMADE KITS

In olden days home remedies included burnt toast. This took the place of activated charcoal, but the fact is that the absorptive powers of burnt toast are so low that they are

nullified by the few chemical impurities in the concoction itself, before reaching the poison in the stomach. As we know, a special process is required to make the real thing. Many authorities recommend buying a small quantity of activated charcoal from industrial suppliers. The author had the trying experience of attempting to buy a mere pound (half a kilogram) of activated charcoal recently. The fact of the matter is that industrial firms will not be tempted by the private sale of an ounce or a pound. Few of the local pharmacies will package and sell activated charcoal as such. So the antidote kits represent the best and easiest solution for obtaining activated charcoal.

SYRUP OF IPECAC

Two things should be in every home, especially where small children abound: an antidote kit and a one ounce (25 gram) bottle of syrup of ipecac. When purchasing ipecac it is necessary to specify *syrup* of ipecac because it comes in other forms and in various concentrations. The one ounce bottle recommended for the home emergency kit—charcoal and ipecac—are standard items in any pharmacy. Even if a doctor is called first during an emergency his instructions may include the use of ipecac to induce throwing up. Having it on hand will save precious time.

Ipecac (*Cephaelis ipecacuanha*) is by no means a new wonder drug. It was introduced to civilization by William Piso (1563–1636). He learned of it from the Brazilian Indians who used it to cure dysentery and several other jungle maladies. The Indians used it also for the same reason it is used in poison emergencies—to cause the victim to throw up. It works because the roots of the ipecac shrub have a product in them called emetine. The product we use is the dry powdered jungle root (the shrub from which these roots are obtained grows only in a steamy hot jungle environment).

145

Poison Control Centers of the United States

Between the ages of one and forty-four, accidents head the list of causes of disability and death. Infants and young children are particularly prone to accidents of all sorts, and accidental poisoning, especially with household chemicals, reached epidemic proportions in the 1950's. The American Academy of Pediatrics recognized the special plight of young children and appointed a panel to study the problem. They discovered that there was no single source of information on the toxic substances in the 250,000 different trade-name products on the market in the United States, despite frequent requests from pediatricians all over the country who needed this information, often in emergency situations. In response Dr. Edward Press, together with several other interested pediatricians, the Evanston, Illinois Health Department and seven Chicago hospitals pooled their resources in the fall of 1953 and established the first Poison Information Center.

The Center consisted of a desk, a telephone, a clerk and files. It reached out to industry to compile information on the ingredients of industrial products, including the extent to which they might be poisonous. They also attempted to establish effective programs for treatment. Out of this effort came a major reference work on the subject which became a mainstay of pediatricians nationwide.

The success of the center led to duplication at many other locations, notably in Boston and New York, but for many years there was no working system for co-operation between researchers in order to share information and avoid repetition. The federal government stepped into the picture and created the National Clearinghouse for Poison Control Centers, which has successfully co-ordinated the efforts of the many regional centers and tabulated the experiences of poison prevention workers across the country. The National Clearinghouse, a part of the Food and Drug Administration, has become the leader in providing services to the nation's recognized poison control centers, which now, a quarter of a century later, number 674, with more than 100 in the state of Illinois alone.

As the poison control system developed, centers varied widely in the kind and quality of services offered. Surveys showed that a large percentage of poison control centers handle as few as one call a day, while others handle as many as eighty. Some centers serve populations of only a few thousand people while others serve areas containing several million people. Staffing varied, ranging from a single person near the ringing phone to a complex system of people and responsibilities—clerks, nurses and physicians backed up by clinical toxicologists, pharmacists, veterinarians, botanists and other specialists concerned with a variety of toxic substances. Further, some centers answered questions from the public, while others responded only to health care professionals.

The need for better centers and more reliable service has led to larger centers which serve larger areas, relying on computer technology to provide up-to-the-minute information. There are six satellite computer terminals in the United States, each directly linked to the central files in Baltimore, Maryland. This system has not been set up at all of the regional centers which would benefit from it because of the high cost, but other modern information distribution systems, including the use of microfilm and periodic updates on product contents and poison prevention techniques from the National Clearinghouse, have fulfilled the original goal of the American Academy of Pediatrics, to give doctors the information they need to save lives.

Dr. John J. Crotty, Director of the National Clearinghouse for Poison Control Centers, explained that the statistics which follow are based on reports from Poison Control Centers submitted voluntarily and that therefore there is no guarantee of their validity. During 1973 the Clearinghouse processed 163,500 reports of ingestions from 517 reporting Centers in 45 different states, the District of Columbia, the Canal Zone, Virgin Islands and military bases abroad. The tabulations presented represent the case reports received from these various locations by the Clearinghouse.

NUMBER OF CASES REPORTED AND THEIR
RESPECTIVE AGE GROUPS, U.S. (1973)

Age Group	Total Number of Cases
0–1	5,837
1	30,400
2	40,680
3	18,086
4	6,673
5–9	6,189
10–14	4,437
15–24	19,394
25–44	14,490
45–64	4,477
More than 64	1,097
Unknown	11,740
Total: All Ages	163,500

PROJECTIONS TOWARD THE FUTURE

From 1950 to the present efforts have been made to prevent poisoning. They include distribution of syrup of ipecac, the institution of child-resistant packaging and a wide variety of educational programs aimed at a number of different audiences: preschool children, young school-age children, parenting classes, parents, health professionals and para-professionals. The fact that "something" is working is reflected in the marked decrease in serious poisoning of children under 5.

Hospitalization is required in less than half the cases and deaths have been reduced from 400 each year in the 1960's to less than 140 in 1975.

Despite a *decrease* in the number of deaths from accidental poisoning of children under 5 years of age there has been a distressing *increase* in total deaths from poisoning in the United States during the last 5 years. This has been most pronounced in the 15 to 24 year age group. During the next 25 years there will be a greater emphasis on setting up Regional Poison Information Centers, on the development of national standards for centers and more effective ways of reducing truly *accidental* poisoning. Improved and more rapid diagnosis of poisonings from unknown toxic substances will result in more precise and efficient handling and a corresponding decrease in death and debility.

ACCIDENTAL INGESTIONS AMONG CHILDREN UNDER 5 YEARS OF AGE, U.S. (1973)

Type of Substance	Number of Cases	% Total
Medicines	52,113	44.3
*Internal	42,215	35.9
*Aspirin	7,763	6.6
*Other	34,452	29.3
*External	9,898	8.4
Cleaning & Polishing Agents	19,132	16.3
Petroleum Products	4,974	4.2
Cosmetics	10,362	8.8
Pesticides	5,591	4.8
Gases	140	0.1
Plants	7,032	6.0
Turpentine, Paints, etc.	6,988	5.9
Miscellaneous	10,517	9.0
Not Specified	740	0.6
Total	117,589	100.0

*These totals are included in Medicines

The problem of non-accidental poisoning may well increase with the rising tempo of stress in an increasingly technological society. Yet those who are poisoned will receive proper care sooner and will be more likely to survive and return to society alive and in a less damaged condition than today. The non-accidental poisoning is a *special* problem that reflects a more serious disorder—a disorder beyond the ability of medical treatment to correct or prevent.

Poisons Information Centres in the United Kingdom

There are no poison control centres in the United Kingdom. Instead there is the closely related Poisons Information Centre. The main difference is that the Poisons Information Centres do not give information to members of the public but only to medical practitioners and Poison Treatment Centres.

By 1963 there were a number of Poisons Information Centres in England but at this time the Standing Medical Advisory Committee prepared a report on the emergency treatment (in hospitals) of cases of acute poisoning and as a result recommended that National Centres be established in London, Cardiff (Wales), Edinburgh (Scotland) and Belfast (Northern Ireland). The objective was to ensure uniform and up-to-date advice from the central files compiled with the full co-operation of many different kinds of industrial organizations.

These national centres are manned on a 24-hour basis and appear to provide a highly satisfactory service. Moreover, it's more economical than maintaining detailed local registers, which are expensive to staff and maintain.

The Poisons Information Centres, however, are not the only sources of information about poisons. The Department has always advised larger hospitals to hold standard works of reference on poisons and to compile their own files of poisonous substances—substances which according to their experience are encountered fairly often. The National Centres are primarily available to back up local knowledge and to provide information about substances less frequently encountered in practice.

The number of calls to Poisons Information Centres has risen (very approximately) at the rate of 2000 each year. This is a reflection of increasing service, matched pretty well in other countries of the world.

Most calls come from hospital doctors and far fewer from general practitioners. Most problems arise over drugs and household products, the remainder being a distinct minority. Most serious and fatal accidents involve drugs and medicines prescribed by doctors rather than "over-the-counter" types. Two thirds of the patients about whom this emergency advice is sought are children, so it appears that potent drugs are frequently left about the house within easy reach of youngsters.

CALLS TO NATIONAL POISONS INFORMATION
SERVICE, U.K. (1975)

Total	20,901
Plants	1,572
Household	5,795
Agriculture	1,342
Industrial	573
Drugs	10,972
Miscellaneous	647

What are the substances involved in most of the emergencies? High on the list are the most intensively promoted mind-affecting drugs. (This is one of the main reasons for insisting that the service be kept up to date.) The older barbiturates, however, are still important. On the other hand, oral contraceptives, which involve so many calls about children, are virtually harmless, even in large single overdoses. The deter-

151

gents, bleaches, perfumes, cosmetics and other household products rarely cause any serious trouble, probably because the amounts are usually small. Yet there are substances that can cause a great deal of harm, for example, paint strippers and solvents of all kinds. And small children it seems often get into products which serve as inhalants and liniments. These can be disastrous. Farm and garden chemicals have a high safety record in England, probably because the official (but voluntary) regulations are so effective.

The Poisons Control Division of Melbourne, Victoria, Australia

Australia doesn't have centres which combine information and treatment—as American Poison Control Centers do, but Poisons *Information* Centres do exist. Victoria's began on August 13, 1962. It was the first such centre in Australia. Poison victims obtain the necessary treatment in hospitals. On request the information centres advise doctors and the public regarding treatment. This is usually done by telephone but doctors particularly may call in person, as the information centres are situated in one or another of the large teaching hospitals. Even so, the information centres are quite independent and as far as J. Ross, the Senior Poisons Control Officer is aware, they are in no way looked upon in any Australian State or Territory as comprising poison control centres, where information and treatment are available.

The Information Centre is usually associated with the "Poisons Division" which is a Division of the Victoria Health Department. Poisons Division Officers are responsible to the Chief Health Officer for most matters relating to the Poisons Act of 1962. This is an Act of Parliament which in Victoria controls the manufacture, sale and possession of dangerous drugs and poisons. It is basically designed to protect the public and those persons exposed to poisons through their occupations.

Poisons used in Victoria are under continuous scrutiny by the Division. These include industrial poisons, household poisons and poisons used in agriculture, scientific research, education and medicine. All such poisons are required by regulation to be properly packaged and labelled and to be handled by persons qualified to do so safely. Officer Ross says that "at the present time occupational and accidental poisonings are relatively unimportant causes of mortality in Victoria. The fact that this position has improved in recent decades in the face of an ever-increasing array of dangerous poisons is the best evidence of the continuing importance of poisons control to community health."

The Poisons Information Centres of South Australia

The Adelaide Children's Hospital is the principal Poisons Information Centre of South Australia. It was officially established by the cabinet and announced by the Minister of Health in 1966.

The first input of information came from the National Register prepared by the Commonwealth Department of Health. The Poisons Register is an index to all types of commercial products with details of their toxic ingredients, their toxic effects and recommended treatment. There are also sections on diagnosis and treatment, special groups of chemicals and general classes of preparations. This information was also used to prepare a National Poisons Register Manual and shorter versions suitable for distribution to hospitals throughout the region.

The Adelaide Children's Hospital serves as the principal poisons information centre in the state but other major hospitals act as information centres too. Each supplies information on all aspects of accidental poisoning as a 24 hour a day service.

Poisons Information Centres provide information available from the Register to

- doctors (regarding the nature of poisons, the antidote if available and the recommended treatment)
- pharmacists (the nature of the poison, emergency or first aid treatment) and
- the public (the need for medical care and first aid).

The details in the Poisons Register and Manual are based on information obtained in confidence from manufacturers and, to preserve this confidence, advice concerning the ingredients of the various products is given only to physicians dealing with a particular case of poisoning.

The Centres also collect information on poisons and poisoning cases. In effect this keeps the Register and Manual up to date.

Most cases of poisoning involve children. This is why the Adelaide Children's Hospital was chosen as the central reference site.

ADELAIDE CHILDREN'S HOSPITAL POISONING STATISTICS	
Categories	Cases Treated: 1974–1975
Internal Medicinals	491
External Medicinals	42
Cosmetics	31
Household products	121
Solvents (non-petroleum)	5
Petroleum distillates	95
Pesticides, agricultural & veterinary	77
Plants	27
Gases and fumes	3
Noxious foodstuffs	7
Miscellaneous	52
Animal hazards	29

```
ADELAIDE CHILDREN'S HOSPITAL POISONING
         STATISTICS 1974-1975
Ages                    Cases Treated
                     Boys            Girls
Under 1 year          21              28
1 to 2 years         183             125
2 to 3 years         166             130
3 to 4 years          79              68
4 to 5 years          30              29
5 to 9 years          45              29
9 to 16 years         23              24
                     ___             ___
     Totals          547             433
```

```
     ADELAIDE CHILDREN'S HOSPITAL
        TELEPHONE INQUIRIES
1975     2,600        1971     1,710
1974     2,368        1970     1,002
1973     2,313        1969       816
1972     2,140        1968       469
```

New Zealand and the Poisons Act

New Zealand exercises control of the advertising, distribution, use, labelling and packaging of all poisons by law: the Poisons Act of 1960 and its Amendments. Control is established through a Poisons Committee created by the Act itself and through a person with the title Registrar of Poisons, whose appointment is authorized by the Act. The Poisons Act and the Amendments made since 1960 comprise a quite lengthy document which spells out definitions, rules and procedures.

Most of the Act details the legal requirements for the sale and custody of poisons, the importation, transportation, storage, labelling and handling of them, including radioactive poisons. The objective is to *prevent* poisoning through the administration of the Act, rather than to provide services in the actual event of poisoning.

The Swiss Poison Information Center

This center gives the same basic services as other poison control centers, providing day and night information on poisoning in man (and animals) by drugs and other chemicals. This includes an identification of the causing agent, its toxicity and the symptoms and recommended treatment.

The Center has many features which are common to other National Information Centers. Information is gathered from the case reports of physicians, from formulas of products (Swiss law requires manufacturers to provide this information), from literature and scientific laboratories, and made available to scientific journals, university professors, poison prevention workers, the mass media for popular education and to manufacturers interested in the prevention of poisoning among their employees.

Dr. A. Abei, Director of the Federal Poisons Office, believes that there are other activities and features probably *not* common to most other Centers of Poison Information.

- There is always an expert physician in charge and at the telephone. When necessary he can obtain the help of consultants by radio.
- When a case history is not available from the poison victim, diagnosis can be established by analysis of clinical signs and symptoms, made possible by a self-developed punched-card system.
- Information is given in German, French, Italian and English.
- An antidote kit, assembled by the Center experts, is supplied to every pharmacy in the country.
- Stored documents are continually updated by information specialists (up to 50 essential contributions daily).

- When not handling emergency calls, medical staff members devote their time exclusively to preparation of a better documentation.
- Files on human poisoning include some 50,000 detailed reports from physicians.
- World-wide literature is available instantly through a computer terminal.
- Expertise in various fields of toxicology is available.
- Federal authorities and manufacturers are informed about all cases of severe poisoning. In return they communicate formulas of products to the Center.

These not-so-common features are the result of sponsorship by various special groups—namely the Swiss Association of Pharmacists, the Swiss Chemical Industries, various government agencies, the University of Zurich, the Accidents Insurance of Switzerland and a host of private individuals.

SWISS POISON INFORMATION CENTER— NUMBER OF INQUIRIES			
1975	12,928	1970	8,651
1974	12,010	1969	7,125
1973	11,416	1968	5,775
1972	10,512	1967	4,665
1971	9,771	1966	1,923

The Dutch National Poison Control Center

The Dutch National Poison Information Center in the Netherlands was formed 13 years ago as a subdivision of the Government Institute of Public Health. This institute collects information from the world's toxicological literature, adds new data of its own, establishes a card index and houses pharmaceutical, toxicological, and many other kinds of laboratory facilities.

Telephone service is given to physicians and pharmaceutical chemists day and night, and of the 8559 calls serviced in 1975, 7729 were for physicians, 216 for pharmacists, 231 for veterinarians and 111 from family doctors. A file of index cards makes fast answers possible. Only in very rare cases is information given to the public. The reason provided by Professor Dr. A. N. P. Heijst, Head of the National Poison Control Center, is that "We are able to offer ourselves this privilege because we live in a small country where a physician or hospital can always be found in close surroundings." A patient who is poisoned can be cured with little delay. Moreover, if he is afflicted with an illness that is mistaken for poison by the family or others, this too can be taken into account and be dealt with efficiently.

DUTCH NATIONAL POISON INFORMATION CENTER—NUMBER OF INQUIRIES

1975	8,559	1969	2,217
1974	7,717	1968	1,729
1973	6,657	1967	1,243
1972	5,453	1966	805
1971	4,233	1965	663
1970	3,030	1964	523

Information at the Center is built up in part by physicians who call there. Physicians are asked to complete questionnaires and return brief accounts of the case, such as the age and sex of the patient, the amount of poison involved, the symptoms and the outcome.

Professor Heijst believes that statistics from the Center don't differ much from those of other nations, but there are a few problems that arise out of special Dutch circumstances. As in most nations around the world, for example, poisoning in children occurs most frequently at the age of two and it happens to boys more often than girls. Most of the compounds involved are household products and of these mainly petroleum distillates and corrosive liquids. Poisoning in adults is usually a matter of self poisoning and is most frequent among young women between the ages of 20 and 30. The greatest number of poisonings occur with barbiturates, not tranquillizers. This, however, may be a typically Dutch problem, for a few years ago the sale of sleeping tablets was prohibited. Following this the poisonings from barbiturates decreased and those of the drug seco-brallobarbital and one called hydroxyzine (prescribed by physicians) increased. This was most unfortunate since barbiturate poisoning was easy to deal with whereas poisonings by the latter two drugs mentioned are more deadly and hard to treat.

DUTCH NATIONAL POISON INFORMATION CENTER—PRODUCTS INVOLVED, 1975

Pharmaceuticals	4,108
Household Chemicals	2,432
Agricultural Products	570
Plants	311
Gases	172
Industrial Poisoning	159
Miscellaneous	231
Total (Approximate)	7,983

REANIMATION CENTER OF THE UNIVERSITY HOSPITAL OF UTRECHT

Information regarding poisons is given to the National Poison Control Center by the Reanimation Center of the University Hospital of Utrecht. (The Hospital is located within walking distance of the Center.) Yearly 900 patients are admitted and of these some 500 are admitted for definite symptoms of poisoning. The Reanimation Center is actually an intensive care unit serviced day and night by 4 physicians (working alternately) and with facilities for heart monitoring, artificial respiration and blood purification. In addition it is associated with a marvelously equipped laboratory for the analysis of poisons and pharmaceuticals.

The whole set-up of the organization, believes Professor Heijst (who heads both the Information Center and the Hospital), fulfills the three essentials of *any* "optimally functioning" Poison Control Center. It

- has centralized information with day and night care
- has people who are actively engaged in poisons work and the treatment of patients in an intensive care department
- has research facilities of a diversified nature as well as the type best suited for specialization in poisons research.

Antidotes, Action and Treatment

This chapter applies pretty well to all four corners of the world. In the event of poisoning the best bet is to contact the nearest Poison Control or Poison Information Center, directly or through a local physician, pharmacist or hospital emergency room. Communication is remarkably swift and up-to-date facts and instructions are only seconds away by phone. When closeness to outside help is a problem, as it might be in the deep country, an antidote kit and simple first aid is the first step. More detailed instructions are available for special interest groups: for hikers in snake-country for instance. This chapter is divided into three parts:

- Household Poisons
- Poisonous Plants
- Poisonous Animals

Charts and tables provide detailed coverage for each part.

Household Poisons

Accidental poisoning is the leading cause of deaths in the home (the number one killer of persons below the age of forty-four). The prime season is winter, when colds and flu run rampant, for during this time medicines—especially pain killers and sedatives—abound and the tendency to misuse them is greatest. Add to this the strange role of alcohol and the effects worsen. Alcohol multiplies the effect of these depressant drugs by four to five times; that is, 400 to 500 per cent.

Prime poison time is Sunday.

A rather horrid fact is that hungry children will eat poisons. And one of the most likely times when children are both hungry and left alone is on Sunday, when parents often sleep late. Then too a child may find a few unattended moments when meals are being prepared. The prime daily danger hours for children are between 4 and 6 P.M. This conclusion came from the Poison Control Center of New York following a survey of 119 hospital emergency rooms. These are the hours when fatigued parents may take a moment to relax or when dinner is on the way and end-of-the-day chores are being squeezed in. There are many moments when children are left to their own often devious devices.

Accidents unfold from the most innocent of circumstances at *all* hours of the day. They don't especially need prime seasons, days or hours. Sometime during the day, for instance, the phone rings. Mother goes to answer it and leaves a bottle of lemon-scented furniture polish open for her daughter to sample. That situations like this happen, on the average, more often than once every three minutes we can be sure, for once every three minutes, on the average, in the United States alone, a serious case of poisoning is logged in by the National Clearing-house for Poison Control Centers. And we can be equally sure that untold numbers of poisoning cases go both unrecognized as poisonings and unreported.

ABOUT THE CHART AND TABLES

FIRST AID FOR POISONING covers the action required most briefly, while POISON HELP! goes into greater detail. The table of CHEMICAL POISONS covers household dangers most comprehensively.

FIRST AID FOR
POISONING

In ALL cases it is important to get the poison out or to dilute the poison. REMEMBER – If anyone swallows poison it is an emergency. (Any non-food substance is a potential poison). Always call for help promptly.

CALL YOUR PHYSICIAN OR POISON CENTER PROMPTLY

SWALLOWED POISONS

1. Make patient vomit, if so directed, **BUT NOT IF:**
   - Patient is unconscious or is having fits.
   - Swallowed poison is a strong corrosive such as acid or lye. Give liquids.
   - Swallowed poison contains kerosene, gasoline, lighter fluid, furniture polish or other petroleum distillates (unless it contains dangerous insecticides as well, which must be removed). Give liquids.

2. Directions for making patient vomit (if physician orders):
   - Give one tablespoonful (one-half ounce) of Syrup of Ipecac for child one (1) year of age, plus at least one cup of water. If no vomiting occurs after 20 minutes, this dose may be repeated one time only.
   - If no Syrup of Ipecac is available, give water and then try to make patient vomit by gently tickling back of throat with spoon or similar blunt object. Place patient in spanking position when vomiting begins.

3. Do not waste time waiting for vomiting, but transport patient, if indicated, to a medical facility. Bring package or container with intact label and any vomited material.

EYE OR SKIN CONTACT — Wash thoroughly with tap water.

INHALATION — Remove from exposure to fumes.

CALL FOR HELP PROMPTLY

Be sure to have 1 oz. Syrup of Ipecac in your home
(Use only on advice of your physician)

Courtesy: John J. Crotty, Director; National Clearinghouse for Poison Control Centers

Poison Help!

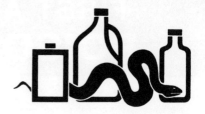

PRODUCT	DO NOT VOMIT	INDUCE VOMITING	SPECIAL INSTRUCTIONS
COSMETICS			
After-Shave Lotions		X	Vomiting not always necessary, call Poison Control Center
Bath Oils		X	Call Poison Control Center
Colognes & Perfumes		X	Call Poison Control Center
Deodorants		X	
Hair Rinse	X		
Hair Straighteners & Permanent Solutions		X	Give citrus juice first, then induce vomiting.
Hand Lotion	X		
Lipstick	X		
Liquid Make-up	X		
Nail Polish & Removers		X	
Shampoo	X		
DRUGS			
Acetominophen		X	Call Poison Control Center
Aspirin Containing Medications		X	
Cold & Cough Medicines		X	
Iron Medicines		X	
Heart Medications		X	Seek medical attention
Sleeping Pills & Tranquillizers		X	Seek medical attention
Vitamins		X	Vomiting not always necessary, call Poison Control Center
TOPICAL MEDICINES			
Diaper Ointments	X		
Hydrogen Peroxide	X		Give milk to drink
Liniments & Oil of Wintergreen		X	Seek *emergency* medical aid
Mercurochrome		X	Vomiting not always necessary, call Poison Control Center

PRODUCT	DO NOT VOMIT	INDUCE VOMITING	SPECIAL INSTRUCTIONS
HOUSEHOLD PRODUCTS			
Adhesives & Glue	X		Call Poison Control Center
Ammonia (Household)	X		Seek *emergency* medical aid
Bleach	X		Give milk to drink
Dishwasher Detergent	X		Seek *emergency* medical aid
Drain Cleaners (Lye)	X		Seek *emergency* medical aid
Fabric Softeners		X	Give milk *before* vomiting
Floor Polishes & Solid Waxes	X		Give milk
Furniture Polish	X		Seek medical attention
Gasoline, Turpentine, Mineral Spirits, Lighter Fluids, etc.	X		Seek medical attention
INSECTICIDES			
Many contain arsenic, lead, organophosphates, petroleum products, etc.		X	Seek *emergency* medical aid
RAT POISON			
May contain boric acid, warfarin, etc. DO NOT VOMIT if strychnine is present		X	Call Poison Control Center
MUSHROOMS		X	Call Poison Control Center
PLANTS		X	Call Poison Control Center

GENERAL INSTRUCTIONS

TO INDUCE VOMITING: Give 3 teaspoons of Syrup of Ipecac, follow with a glass or more of warm water and repeat in 15 minutes if vomiting has not occurred. DO NOT GIVE SALT WATER.

HOWEVER Vomiting is not recommended in all cases and may not be necessary in some cases. Before emergency measures have been taken, always try to reach your Poison Control Center or physician.

REMEMBER: When necessary to seek medical attention, take the poison container with label intact to treatment facility.

Courtesy of the Poison Control Center at Grady Memorial Hospital, Atlanta, Georgia 30303. (Supplied by the Atlanta Association of Independent Insurance Agents)

Table of Chemical Poisons

Chemical Poison	Chief Signs and Symptoms	Emergency Treatment
Acetone Nail polish remover Paint and varnish remover	Nausea, vomiting, decreased pulse, difficulty in breathing, irritation to kidneys, stupor.	After patient has vomited, give stimulants such as strong coffee or tea.
Acids Acetic Hydrochloric (muriatic) Nitric Phosphoric Sulphuric	Corrosion of membranes of the mouth and throat and esophagus. Vomiting, intense pain, collapse. Feeble heart beat, rapid pulse.	Give liberal doses of milk of magnesia, milk, soapy water, or egg whites.
Alkalies Sodium hydroxide (lye, caustic soda) Potassium hydroxide (caustic potash) "Saniflush," etc.	Corrosion of mucous membranes of the digestive tract. Vomiting. Intense pain. Feeble heart beat. Rapid pulse. Blood often present in vomit and in stools.	Give strong solution of vinegar or citrus juice followed by olive oil, melted butter, or other nontoxic oil. Do not induce vomiting.
Alcohol, Methyl Wood alcohol Paint or shellac thinner	Depression, muscle inco-ordination, headache, disturbed vision, nausea, blindness, delirium, collapse; often fatal.	After patient has vomited, give large dose of baking soda followed by a dose of epsom salts. Have the patient inhale spirits of ammonia if available.
Amyl acetate Nail polish remover Banana oil Pear oil Lacquer thinner	Irritation of eyes, coughing, abdominal pain, vomiting, respiratory difficulty.	Give strong stimulants such as coffee or tea. Do not give patient anything to make him vomit.

Poison	Symptoms	Treatment
Arsenic Fly paper Fowler's solution Paris green Lead arsenate Ant or rat poison	Metallic taste, burning pain in esophagus or stomach, vomiting and diarrhea, thirst, choking sensation, garlic odor on breath, cold skin, rapid weak pulse, collapse, convulsions, coma.	Give strong stimulants, followed by castor oil or epsom salts.
Barbiturates Barbital Phenobarbital Seconal Nembutal Amytal Pentothal	Small doses produce sleep. Large doses produce headache, mental confusion, coma, blue lips and fingernails, dilated pupils, slow or irregular breathing.	Administer strong stimulants. If breathing remains normal, patient will probably sleep off the effects of the drug.
Benzene, Benzol Toluene Xylol Floor wax or polish Some shoe polish	Nausea, vomiting, headache, irregular pulse, dizziness, excitement, depression, coma. Heart failure. Damage to blood-forming organs.	Give large amounts of vegetable (cooking) oil, not mineral oil.
Benzine Gasoline Kerosene Petroleum ether Cleaner's naphtha	Inhalation produces cyanosis, flushed face, coma, dilated pupils and respiratory failure. Swallowing produces burning of mouth, nausea, vomiting, drunkenness, thirst, slow pulse, difficult breathing, convulsions and coma.	Do not induce vomiting. Give large amounts of vegetable (cooking) oil, not mineral oil.
LSD d-lysergic acid diethylamide	Dilated pupils, exhilaration or extreme anxiety, delirium, muscle cramps, inability to move, convulsions.	Administer tranquillizers (chlorpromazine), and reassure the patient. Do not restrain physically.

167

Chemical Poison	Chief Signs and Symptoms	Emergency Treatment
Carbon monoxide Coal gas Automobile exhaust	Dizziness, weakness, headache, stupor, throbbing pulse, increased blood pressure, skin dusky, lips pink, paralysis, coma.	Remove patient to fresh air and begin artificial respiration. Protect from shock.
Carbon tetrachloride Noninflammable cleaning fluid Fire extinguisher fluid	Headache, drowsiness, confusion, coma. Abdominal pain, dilated pupils. Kidney and liver damage follows acute symptoms.	Give strong coffee or tea in addition to the treatment listed below for induction of vomiting and prevention of shock.
Chlorine Sodium hypochlorite Bleaching solution of "Clorox" type	Inhalation produces irritation of the lungs and eyes, spasmlike cough, choking, vomiting, cyanosis, collapse. Swallowing produces irritation of the gastrointestinal tract and extreme pain.	If inhaled, remove patient to fresh air, give artificial respiration, and have the patient inhale spirits of ammonia. If swallowed, treat as listed below for production of vomiting and prevention of shock.
Copper salts Copper sulphate Blue stone Blue vitriol Zinc salts	Nausea, vomiting, purging, severe abdominal pains, cold clammy skin, delirium, coma, convulsions.	The patient should vomit repeatedly. Then, give egg white of magnesia followed by strong coffee or tea.
Cyanides Hydrocyanic acid Cyanogen Some insect poison Gopher poison	Large doses produce instant death. Small doses cause vomiting, diarrhea, difficult breathing, glassy eyes, pale face, blood-stained foam on mouth, stupor, coma.	After patient has vomited, give dose of hydrogen peroxide.

168

Fluorides
Cockroach or insect poison

Nausea, vomiting, abdominal cramps, weakness, fall in blood pressure, deep rapid respiration, convulsions, coma.

Give calcium tablets, lime water, chalk, or milk.

Formaldehyde
Home disinfectant
Preserving fluid for natural history specimens

Swallowing produces irritation of mouth and gut. Irritation of lungs. Severe abdominal pain, nausea, vomiting, rapid pulse, blood in urine. Intense irritation of eyes and lungs upon breathing fumes.

Before having patient vomit, give him dilute ammonia water, egg whites, or milk. After he has vomited, give large doses of baking soda in water.

Iodine
Tincture of iodine
Iodex salve
Lugol's solution

Brown color on lips and mouth. Burning pain in stomach, vomiting. Bloody purging, heart depression, cold skin, convulsions, collapse.

Give large quantities of starch (bread, flour, corn starch, etc.) followed by strong coffee or tea.

Lead
Red lead
White lead
Paints

Pain in stomach, thirst, blood in stools and vomit, weakness, paralysis, convulsions, collapse.

After patient has vomited, give him calcium tablets, powdered chalk, or milk followed by epsom salts.

Mercury
Bichloride of mercury
Corrosive sublimate

Severe pain in mouth, throat, stomach, increase in saliva, blood and mucus in vomit. Watery bloody diarrhea, followed in 1 or 2 days by inflammation of colon, blood in urine, coma, collapse.

Give egg whites immediately.

Chemical Poison	Chief Signs and Symptoms	Emergency Treatment
Opium Codeine Heroin Laudanum Morphine	Mental exhilaration followed by drowsiness. Pupils of eyes pinpoint. Slow shallow breathing, slow onset of unconsciousness, muscles relaxed, skin pale, cold sweat, blue lips, irregular breathing.	After patient has vomited, give him a dose of charcoal and aluminum hydroxide. Follow this with strong coffee or tea, and keep the patient awake and warm until a physician arrives.
Phenols Carbolic acid Creosote Lysol	Burning pain from mouth to stomach, white patches in mouth, depression, weakness, nausea. Blood in urine, fall in body temperature. Pale, livid, clammy face.	Give patient large quantities of any nontoxic oil (olive oil, mineral oil, cooking oil, etc.). Also give lime water and egg whites. Do not give patient anything to make him vomit.
Phosphorous Matches Rat poison (read label)	Gastrointestinal pain, garlic odor, vomiting of blood, bloody diarrhea. If patient survives, remission of symptoms in 2 to 3 days. Later symptoms: skin eruption, enlarged liver, jaundice, pulse weak, heart weak, convulsions.	Give large amounts of mineral oil, followed by epsom salts.

In every type of poisoning, immediate medical aid is essential. Further, vomiting should be induced if the poison is swallowed (except in those cases noted where it is contraindicated) by causing the patient to gag or by administration of warm soapy water or a tartar emetic. Every patient must be kept warm until the physician arrives, and other standard means to combat shock should be instituted. Should the patient cease breathing before medical aid is available, artificial respiration should be given.

From *The Book of Health* edited by Randolph Clark and Russell Cumley, © 1973 by Litton Educational Publishing, Inc. Reprinted by permission of Van Nostrand Reinhold Company.

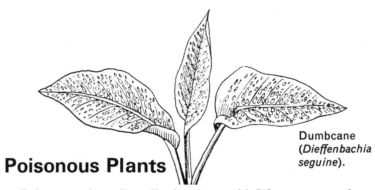

Dumbcane
(*Dieffenbachia seguine*).

Poisonous Plants

Poisonous plants literally dot the world. We encounter them in the house, the flower and vegetable gardens, in meadows, fields and swamps and many moist places in the warmer regions of the world. In addition, we encounter them as ornamental plants, trees and shrubs in the yard or along road-sides and in the deepest wilds. The following table covers them as they appear over most of the world.

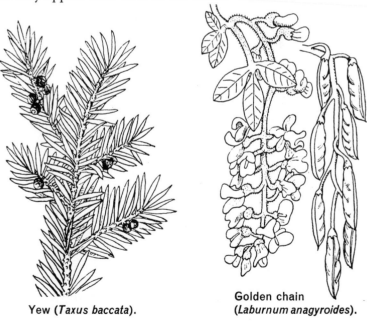

Yew (*Taxus baccata*).

Golden chain
(*Laburnum anagyroides*).

Poisonous Plants

Name	Part of Plant	Active Principle	Symptoms and Treatment
		HOUSE PLANTS	
Hyacinth *Hyacinthus orientalis*	Bulb		Intense digestive upset.
Narcissus or daffodil *Narcissus* sps.	Bulb	Toxic alkaloids (?)	Severe gastroenteritis, vomiting, diarrhea, trembling, convulsions.
Oleander *Nerium oleander*	All parts, green or dry. Food skewered on oleander branches becomes poisonous. Single leaf is said to be lethal.	Cardiac glycosides: oleandroside, oleandrin, nerioside	Nausea, depression, lowered and irregular pulse, mydriasis, bloody diarrhea, paralysis, death. Atropine, emetics, gastric lavage, and symptomatic medication. Can produce dermatitis.
Poinsettia *Euphorbia pulcherrima*	Juice of leaves, stems, flowers, or fruit; green or dry	Various toxins in the acrid milky sap	Intense emesis, abdominal pains, diarrhea, delirium. Sap causes dermatitis externally and temporary blindness if rubbed in eyes. Use demulcents, intestinal astringents, gastric sedatives, CNS and circulatory stimulants.
Mistletoe *Phoradendron flavescens* (American) and *Viscum album* (European)	Berries	Beta-phenylethylamine and tyramine	Several deaths among children have been attributed to eating the berries. Tea brewed from berries has caused fatality. Death occurred about 10 hours after symptoms of acute gastroenteritis and cardiovascular collapse. Treatment symptomatic.
Rosary pea, Crabseye, precatory bean, jequirity bean *Abrus precatorius*	Seeds	The phytotoxin abrin and the tetanic glycoside abric acid	Extremely toxic. Symptoms resemble tetanus or typhoid. Nausea, vomiting, severe diarrhea, weakness, cold perspiration, colic, weak and accelerated pulse, and trembling of hands. Use saline purgative and symptomatic treatment.

Plant	Parts	Toxin	Symptoms and Treatment
Castor bean *Ricinus communis*	All parts, mainly seeds	The phytotoxin ricin	Produces burning sensation in mouth and throat. Two to four seeds may produce serious poisoning, about eight seeds considered lethal. Symptoms include nausea, vomiting, violent purging, bloody diarrhea, and dullness of vision. Gastric lavage, administration of saline cathartics, maintenance of fluid and electrolyte equilibrium, and symptomatic measures recommended.
Dieffenbachia, Dumbcane *Dieffenbachia seguine* or *picta*	All parts including sap	Calcium oxalate crystals, toxic protein	Ingestion produces rapid irritation, burning of surface of mouth, tongue, and lips, copious salivation, and edematous swelling. May cause death if swelling blocks air passages of throat. Juice may cause intense irritation on skin. Treatment symptomatic, pain relieved with meperidine HCl; aluminum-magnesium hydroxide useful as demulcent and neutralizing agent.

FLOWER GARDEN PLANTS

Plant	Parts	Toxin	Symptoms and Treatment
Larkspur *Delphinium ajacis* and other species	Young plant, seeds	Poisonous alkaloids, mainly delphinine which is a polycyclic diterpene	Ingestion produces digestive upset and symptoms of nervous excitement or depression. May be fatal. Perform gastric lavage and treat for alkaloid poisoning and CNS excitation using short-acting barbiturates because of subsequent depression.
Monkshood *Aconitum napellus* and other species	Roots, seeds, leaves	Poisonous alkaloids, mainly aconitine which is a polycyclic diterpene	Poisonous alkaloids affect vagus nerve from brain causing a slowing of the heart. Other effects include tingling and numbing sensation of the lips and tongue, irregular pulse, dimness of vision, and respiratory failure. Keep victim warm, and in shock position. Treat for alkaloid poisoning. Use gastric lavage and circulatory stimulants if necessary.

Name	Part of Plant	Active Principle	Symptoms and Treatment
Autumn crocus or Meadow saffron *Colchicum autumnale*	All parts, bulbs, seeds	Colchicine alkaloid	Cerebral depression; circulatory collapse, diarrhea, nausea. Treat symptomatically and with activated charcoal.
Star of Bethlehem *Ornithogalum umbellatum*	All parts, bulbs, leaves fresh or dry	Alkaloids	Nausea, nervous symptoms, and general disturbance of the intestinal tract. Treatment symptomatic.
Lily of the valley *Convallaria majalis*	Leaves, flowers, roots	The cardiac glycosides convallarin and convallamarin	Heart stimulation similar to digitalis glycosides. Dizziness and vomiting may occur in 1–2 hours, if large quantities are eaten. See digitalis for treatment.
Iris or Blue Flag *Iris versicolor*	Leaves and root stalks	Acrid resinous substance irisin	Produces severe but not usually serious digestive upset. Acts on GI tract, liver, and pancreas, causing inflammation of the intestinal tract with diarrhea. Can also cause dermatitis. Antidote drugs include antihistaminics, barbiturates, and paregoric.
Foxglove *Digitalis purpurea*	Leaves and seeds	Several glycosides, mainly digitoxin, digitalin, and digitonin	One of the sources of the drug digitalis. In large amounts the active principles cause dangerously irregular heartbeat and pulse, usually digestive upset, and mental confusion. May be fatal. Have patient vomit or perform gastric lavage. Sedative drugs of value to control restlessness. Potassium chloride orally or IV if renal function not impaired; atropine sulfate (2 mg in adults) blocks influence of exaggerated vagal tone. Use procainemide HCl or quinidine sulfate for ventricular tachycardia. See digitalis.

Plant	Poisonous Part	Toxic Principle	Symptoms and Treatment
Bleeding heart (Dutchman's breeches) *Dicentra cucullaria*	Foliage, roots	Several isoquinoline-type alkaloids including apomorphine, protoberberine, and protopine	Symptoms include trembling, staggering, convulsions, and labored breathing. Has proved fatal to livestock. Treatment includes use of cardiac and respiratory stimulants and sedatives.
Christmas rose *Helleborus niger*	Rootstocks and leaves	Two very toxic glycosides, helleborin and helleborein	Diarrhea, gastric distress, and nervous effects. Juice produces skin inflammation and numbing sensations in mouth. Wash skin with soap. Have person vomit and treat for digitalis or aconite poisoning, depending upon symptoms.
Four o'clock *Mirabilis jalapa*	Root, seed	The alkaloid trigonelline	Irritant to skin and mucosa. The alkaloid has a laxative effect. Treatment symptomatic.
Sweet pea *Lathyrus odoratus*	Seeds or peas	Beta (gamma-L-glutamyl)-amino-propionitrile	Large quantities in diet produce paralytic syndrome (lathyrism). Remove from diet. Casein given to animals has protected against paralytic effect.
Morning Glory, (Heavenly Blue, Pearly Gates, Flying Saucers, varieties) *Ipomoea violacea*	Seeds	The clavine alkaloids ergine, isoergine, clymoclavine, and others all chemically related to LSD	From 50–200 powdered seeds ingested are capable of inducing psychotomimetic effects for several hours. Used by thrill-seekers because of LSD-like effects. Produces nausea, uterine stimulation, euphoria. Has produced death by suicide presumably due to CNS effects. Chlorpromazine effective as antidote.

VEGETABLE GARDEN PLANTS

Plant	Poisonous Part	Toxic Principle	Symptoms and Treatment
Rhubarb *Rheum rhaponticum*	Leaf *blade* (not the petiole which is edible)	Oxalic acid	Severe intermittent abdominal pains, vomiting and weakness. Muscular cramps and tetany due to hypocalcemia may occur. Large amounts of raw or cooked leaves can cause convulsions, coma, followed rapidly by death. Give milk or lime water and induce emesis, or use gastric lavage with lime water. Give calcium gluconate 10% IV if tetany or hypocalcemia appears.

Name	Part of Plant	Active Principle	Symptoms and Treatment
Potato *Solanum tuberosum*	Green "sunburned" spots and sprouts of potato tubers, green stems and leaves.	Solanine alkaloids	Cold, clammy skin; nausea; mental confusion; respiratory and cardiac depression. Has caused deaths. Symptomatic treatment.

ORNAMENTAL PLANTS

Name	Part of Plant	Active Principle	Symptoms and Treatment
Daphne *Daphne mezereum* and other species	Berries, bark, leaves	Bitter glycoside daphnin and an acid resinous mixture	Plant intensely acrid, producing vesication when rubbed on skin. Ingestion produces burning sensation in mouth. Vomiting, diarrhea with blood and mucus, stupor, weakness, convulsions, and death. Perform gastric lavage, treat for irritation of GI tract. For pain use meperidine (Demerol).
Wisteria *Wisteria floribunda* (Japanese) and *W. sinensis* (Chinese)	Seeds or pods	Poisonous resin and a glucoside wisterin; flowers are nontoxic	Mild to severe gastroenteritis with repeated vomiting, abdominal pain, and diarrhea. Induce emesis. Once toxic symptoms begin, treatment is symptomatic, using antiemetics (chlorpromazine) and fluid replacement therapy.
Golden chain *Laburnum anagyroides*	Bean-like capsules in which the seeds are suspended	The quinolizidine alkaloid cytisine	Excitement, inco-ordination, vomiting, convulsions, coma, and death through asphyxiation. Considered very poisonous shrub or tree in Britain. Action similar to nicotine. Treat for alkaloid poisoning and symptomatically.
Mountain laurel *Kalmia latifolia* and *augustifolia*	All parts	Andromedotoxin, a resinoid substance	Curare-like effect on skeletal muscle. Stimulation of striated muscle followed by depression. Inhibitory action on heart tissues. Depresses the CNS, causing respiratory failure and ultimately death. Treatment is symptomatic and supportive.

Plant	Poisonous parts	Toxic principle	Symptoms and treatment
Rhododendron, Western azalea *Rhododendron albiflorum, macrophyllum, maximum, occidentale* —(*azalea occidentale*)	All parts	Andromedotoxin	Salivation, lacrimation, rhinitis, vomiting, convulsions, bradycardia, hypotension and paralysis. Treatment, see Veratrum, page 182.
Yellow jessamine *Gelsemium sempervirens*	Whole plant, berries	Toxic alkaloids gelsemine and gelseminine	These alkaloids chiefly depress and paralyze motor nerve endings. Depression of the motor neurons of the brain and spinal cord results in respiratory arrest. Atropine and artificial respiration.
Lantana *Lantana camara*	Berries	A polycyclic triterpenoid named lantadene A	Extreme muscular weakness, gastrointestinal irritation, and circulatory collapse. Syndrome resembles atropine poisoning. Induce vomiting or perform gastric lavage. Treatment, see atropine.
Yew *Taxus baccata* and *T. canadensis*	All parts, especially *seed* if chewed; fleshy red pulp of fruit least harmful	Taxine, an alkaloid	Nausea, vomiting, diarrhea, abdominal pain, circulatory failure, and difficulty in breathing. The alkaloid depresses the heart function. Can cause dermatitis. Induce vomiting, perform gastric lavage, and treat for circulatory failure and alkaloid poisoning.

TREES AND SHRUBS

Plant	Poisonous parts	Toxic principle	Symptoms and treatment
Wild and cultivated cherries *Prunus serotina* (Wild black cherry), *virginiana* (Choke cherry), *pennsylvanica* (Pin cherry)	Twigs, leaves, bark, and fruit stones	Cyanogenitic glycosides including amygdalin, prunasin, etc. which release cyanide when eaten	Difficult breathing, vertigo, convulsions, and coma. A rapid reaction with death usually less than one hour after eating. Treat for cyanide poisoning.

Name	Part of Plant	Active Principle	Symptoms and Treatment
Oaks *Quercus* sps.	Acorns, young shoots, leaves when eaten in large quantities	Tannic acid and a volatile oil	Causes constipation, bloody stools, and gradual kidney damage. Takes a large amount for poisoning. Children should not be allowed to chew on acorns. Saline purgatives to hasten elimination.
Elderberry, Black elder *Sambucus canadensis* and other sps.	Shoots, leaves, bark, roots	Alkaloid and glycoside. Small amounts of hydrocyanic acid are produced under certain conditions	Children have been poisoned by using pieces of the pithy stems for blowguns. Fresh berries essentially harmless. These may produce nausea if too many are eaten. Symptoms include nausea and digestive upset. Treat for cyanide in serious poisoning.
Black locust *Robinia pseudoacacia*	Bark, sprouts, foliage, seeds	The phytotoxin robin and a glycoside robitin	Anorexia, lassitude, weakness, nausea, vomiting, shock, and marked dilation of pupils. Pulse weak and irregular. Death occurs within 2–3 days. Treatment symptomatic.
Bloodroot *Sanguinaria canadensis*	The underground stems, roots, and their red contents	The alkaloid sanguinarine	Causes irritation of the mucous membranes of the mouth, throat, and stomach with intense burning, nausea, and vomiting. If absorbed, alkaloids affect the nervous system, depress the heart, cause coma, and produce temporary paralysis. Induce vomiting, then give warm milk. Perform gastric lavage and treat irritated GI tract. Prevent circulatory collapse.
Poison ivy (Erroneously called poison oak) *Toxicodendron radicans* or *Rhus toxicodendron*	All parts, even the smoke from burning it.	An oil-resin called urushiol which is made up of phenolic substances like 3-n-pentadecylcatechol	Produces a severe allergenic response causing dermatitis upon contact resulting in inflammation, blistering, and vesicles. As skin breaks, a liquid exudes and scabs or crusts form. Combination of oil-resin with skin proteins is immediate and yellow soap only washes off the excess. Treatment topical with lotions and creams for symp-

Plant	Toxic part	Toxic principle	Symptoms and treatment
Poison sumac *Toxicodendron vernix*	As above	As above	tomatic relief. Oral and injectable products of limited value except for corticosteroids in extreme cases. Do not use alcohol or organic solvents on the skin as this will spread the urushiol.

PLANTS IN WOODED AREAS

Plant	Toxic part	Toxic principle	Symptoms and treatment
Jack-in-the-pulpit *Arisaema triphyllum* and other sps.	All parts, especially the rhizome	Needle-like crystals of calcium oxalate	Calcium oxalate crystals become embedded in the mucous membranes of mouth provoking intense irritation and a burning sensation. In large doses may cause gastroenteritis. Seldom fatal. Treatment symptomatic, pain relieved with meperidine HCl; aluminum-magnesium hydroxide useful as demulcent and neutralizing agent.
Moonseed *Menispermum canadense*	Roots and fruit	Bitter alkaloids	Fruits and leaves resemble those of grape vine and thus mistaken for this plant. Contains a single seed. (True grapes contain several small seeds.) The rough sharp ridges of the fruit pits may also cause mechanical injury to the intestines. Has caused death in children. Treatment symptomatic.
Mayapple *Podophyllum peltatum*	Green fruit, foliage, roots	A crude resinous material podophyllin	Ripe fruit (yellow) edible. Green fruit and other parts cause severe diarrhea; gastroenteritis accompanied with vomiting. May also cause dermatitis. Young plant eaten as pot herb has caused human death. Treatment symptomatic.
Baneberry, Snakeberry *Actaea rubra, A. alba,* and *A. spicata*	Berries, rootstock, sap	An essential oil	As few as six berries can cause gastroenteritis, diarrhea, vomiting, and delirium. If absorbed the acrid principles can cause tachycardia and dizziness. Fatalities have been reported. Perform gas-

Name	Part of Plant	Active Principle	Symptoms and Treatment
			tric lavage. Support circulation and treat for gastric inflammation.
Fly agaric mushroom *Amanita muscaria*	All parts	Muscarine	Intense sweating, salivation, wheezing, irregular breathing and heart rate, mental confusion, muscular twitching, possible vomiting, diarrhea, and abdominal pain. Can be fatal within an hour. Induce vomiting, gastric lavage. Treatment for CNS stimulation and dehydration. Atropine is antidote for any poisoning by mushrooms containing muscarine.
Destroying angel, death cup *Amanita phalloides*	All parts	Five related cyclo-peptides, phalloidin, phallion, α, β, γ, amanitin	No symptoms for 6–15 hours, then sudden severe seizure of extreme abdominal pain, vomiting, and diarrhea. Hepatic and renal involvement in 3–4 days. CNS signs are usually terminal. There is no antidote, treatment being symptomatic and supportive. Mortality rate from 50 to 90 per cent. Corticosteroids, broad-spectrum antibiotics, vitamins, C, K, B complex, and dextrose and sodium chloride solutions may be helpful.
Panther mushroom *Amanita pantherina*	All parts	Muscarine	Same as with *Amanita muscaria*
Jack-o'-lantern fungus *Clitocybe illudens* and related species, *C. sud-orifiva* and *C. morbifera*	All parts	Muscarine	Similar to *Amanita muscaria*, but in reported cases no fatalities have occurred. Common symptoms include vomiting, perspiration, and salivation. Treat for muscarine poisoning.
False morels *Helbella esculenta*, *H. gigas*, and *H. underwoodii*	All parts	An unknown proto-plasmic poison	Activity essentially hepatotoxic, with additional effects on the hematopoietic systems and CNS. Has latent period of 6–10 hours between ingestion and symptoms. Fatal poisonings rare in the U.S. Treatment same as with *Amanita phalloides*.

Plant	Part	Toxic agent	Symptoms and treatment
Inky cap *Coprinus atramentarius*	All parts	Unknown	Ingestion of these followed by ingestion of alcohol yields symptoms (in certain individuals) which resemble those of the alcohol-disulfiram (Antabuse) syndrome. Symptoms occur from $\frac{1}{2}$-2 hours after ingestion and include flushing, palpitations, dyspnea, hyperventilation, and tachycardia. Recovery usually spontaneous and complete; however, severe cases may require gastric lavage and symptomatic treatment.

PLANTS IN SWAMP OR MOIST AREAS

Plant	Part	Toxic agent	Symptoms and treatment
Water hemlock (Cowbane) *Cicuta maculata* and other species	All parts, mostly the roots	Resin-like substance, cicutoxin	Symptoms appear in 15 minutes and include severe gastric pain, great mental excitation and frenzy, vomiting, salivation, violent spasmodic convulsions alternating with periods of relaxation. Pupils dilate and delirium is common. Death may occur within 15 minutes after ingestion of a lethal amount. Perform stomach lavage. Control convulsions with parenteral short-acting barbiturates. Use morphine or derivatives if necessary.
Marsh marigold *Caltha palustris*	Top leaves and stems	Protoanemonin, a volatile oil	Irritant sap may cause salivation, inflamed oral mucosa, GI irritation, and diarrhea. Convulsions may occur if ingested in large quantity. When cooked, the "greens" can be eaten without ill effects. Treatment is symptomatic.
Skunk cabbage *Symplocarpus foetidus*	Leaves, rhizomes	Calcium oxalate crystals	Needles of calcium oxalate become embedded in the mucous membranes and produce intense irritation and a burning sensation. Mortality in human beings unknown. Leaves can be eaten if cooked in several waters to which has been added sodium bicarbonate. Treat with demulcents.

181

PLANTS IN FIELDS, MEADOWS, PASTURES, AND ROADSIDES

Name	Part of Plant	Active Principle	Symptoms and Treatment
Green or false hellebore, Indian poke *Veratrum viride*	Roots, leaves and seeds	Mixture of veratrum alkaloids	Salivation, vomiting, sweating, hypotension, muscular weakness, shallow respiration, irregular pulse and bradycardia. Hypothermia, convulsions, and death from asphyxia. Induce emesis, gastric lavage, saline cathartics, support respiration. Use atropine to block reflex bradycardia. Levarterenol or ephedrine used for hypotension. Epinephrine is contraindicated.
Buttercups *Ranunculus abortivus*, *R. acris*, and other sps.	All parts, especially the juice	Ranunculin and protoanemonin	Have vesicant properties. Orally cause salivation, GI irritation, and diarrhea. May cause convulsions if ingested in large quantity. Treatment is symptomatic.
European bittersweet, climbing nightshade *Solanum dulcamara*	Leaves and unripe green fruits	A glycoalkaloid solanine	Ingestion results in burning in the throat, nausea, dizziness, dilation of pupils, convulsions, and general muscular weakness. Other symptoms include GI irritation, anorexia, vomiting, constipation, or diarrhea. Death is result of paralysis, although not all ingestions are fatal. Induce vomiting or use gastric lavage and treat symptomatically.
Black, deadly, or common nightshade *Solanum nigrum*	As above	As above	As above (Ripe berries and young stems and leaves, when cooked, may be edible.)
Horse or bull nettle *Solanum carolinense*	As above	As above	As above (Caused death of 6-year-old child in Delaware County, Pennsylvania, in January of 1963.)

Plant	Toxic parts	Toxin / Symptoms and treatment
Poison hemlock *Conium maculatum*	Leaves, stem, and fruit	Coniine and other related alkaloids	Trembling, ataxia (lower limbs), dilation of pupils, bradycardia, coma, and eventual death through respiratory failure. Perform gastric lavage. Treat symptomatically.
Jimson weed or thornapple *Datura stramonium D. metel, D. metaloides, D. suaveolens,* and other sps.	All parts, especially seeds	The solanaceous alkaloids, atropine, hyoscyamine, and scopolamine	Symptoms include intense thirst, dilated pupils, vomiting, vertigo, dryness of mouth, rapid and weak pulse, partial blindness, excessive thirst, delirium, incoherence; later, slow respiration, hyperthermia, rapid and weak pulse, convulsions or coma preceding death. Handling leaves followed by rubbing eyes can cause dilation of pupils. Wash hands after handling. Treatment, see atropine.
Pokeweed, pigeonberry, inkberry *Phytolacca americana, P. decandra*	Roots and leaves, fruit is least toxic	A resinous material and a water-soluble saponin	Produces burning sensation in mouth, GI cramps, vomiting, diarrhea. Later, visual disturbance, perspiration, salivation, lassitude, prostration, cardiac and respiratory depression. If recovery does not occur in 24 hours, may be fatal. Perform gastric lavage, and treat for circulatory and respiratory depression. Death in a 5-year-old child has been documented.
Dogbane *Apocynum cannabinum* (Indian hemp, dogbane), *A. androsaemifolium* (spreading dogbane)	Green or dry leaves and tops	The resinoid apocynin and glucosides apocynein and cymarin	Increase in temperature, pulse and blood pressure, cold sweating, dilation of pupils, discoloration of mouth, refusal to eat and drink, GI disturbance, finally death. Treatment is symptomatic.
Hemp, marihuana *Cannabis sativa*	Leaves and flowering tops	A resinous mixture of tetrahydro-cannabinols	Individual reaction extremely variable. Generally have period of euphoria and elation followed by a heightened sensitivity to stimulation. This is followed by hallucinations and mental confusion. With heavier doses, depression and comatose

183

sleep follow. Little or no withdrawal symptoms on long use. Effects can be produced by smoking resin-containing parts or ingesting crude resin. Death may occur in overdose due to its cardiac effect. Federal law prohibits (without license) the possession of living or dried cannabis or parts of the plant. Treatment symptomatic. Gastric lavage, CNS, and cardiac stimulants.

Reprinted from the *American Journal of Pharmaceutical Education*, volume 30, by Dr. Ara Der Marderosin, Philadelphia College of Pharmacy and Science, 43rd Street and Kingsessing Avenue, Philadelphia, Pa. 19104, © *American Journal of Pharmaceutical Education* via the American Association of Colleges of Pharmacy.

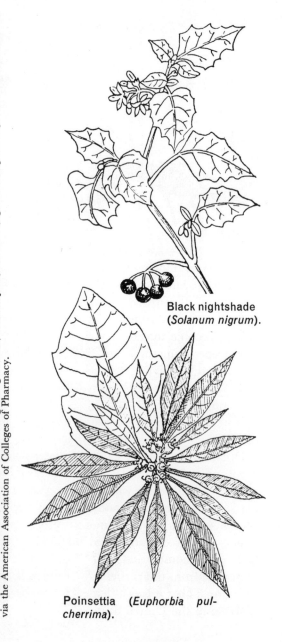

Black nightshade (*Solanum nigrum*).

Poinsettia (*Euphorbia pulcherrima*).

Poisonous Animals

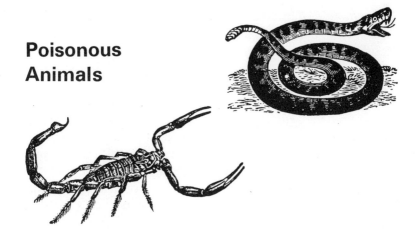

Wild animal bites—from foxes, rabbits, squirrels, chipmunks, monkeys, coyotes, wolves, raccoons and bats—can be dangerous for any or all of three reasons:

- bacteria and other micro-organisms can cause the wound to become infected
- deeper punctures can lead to tetanus (more commonly called "lockjaw")
- if by chance the animal has rabies this too could be transmitted.

Now if the animal is a snake we add a fourth problem, that of venom.

Question One: How can we tell a poisonous snakebite from a non-poisonous one? Usually the venomous types have fangs as well as teeth. The wound will reveal two deep punctures if the snake is venomous and only tiny teeth marks if it isn't. Moreover, bites from venomous beasts usually result in swelling, some pain, discoloration and tingling of the fingertips. It may be a small consolation, but 75% of the bites in the United States are from the rattlesnake—which is easy to recognize by its rattles. (That solves at least three fourths of the identification problem in the United States.)

Question Two: Snakebite victims may be hikers in the great wilds, at least half an hour from the nearest help—what then? Hikers and travellers in snake country would do well to have a snakebite kit on hand, as well as brief but clear instructions on first aid. (For example the wallet-sized instructions provided by one of the world's experts on snakebite—Dr. Herbert Stanke.) Poison Control Centers should be contacted as soon as possible, for they have access to a centralized record on the availability of antivenin. (Zoos usually have antivenin, good against both their common and exotic types of beast.)

In the United States anyone bitten by a rattlesnake is usually given the "polyvalent antitoxin" good against most of the thirty different kinds of rattlers. Antivenin is also available for the other most common types of poisonous North American snakes—the coral, water moccasin and copperhead types.

For poisonous snakes Australia is exceeded by none. The same applies to the research and development of antivenin, and its availability. To date this includes the brown snake, death adder, Malayan cobra, Papuan black snake, sea snake, tiger snake and the taipan.

Antivenin is available over the greater part of the rest of the world. Central and South America have antivenin for the rattler and the bushmaster; Asia, for the cobra, krait and Malayan viper; Africa for the puff adder and mamba; the Indo-Pacific region for the sea snake; Japan for the mamushi and habu and Europe for its only poisonous native snake—the European viper.

Antivenin, in addition, is available for the black widow, red back and other species of spider, the scorpion and the Gila monster.

Antivenins can be single shot devices, aimed at only one species, like the black widow spider or the Arizona scorpion, or they can be multi-shot devices, aimed at two or more species —like the combined tiger snake-taipan snake antivenin (one can be used for the other in an emergency but they are not *ideally* interchangeable). Then too there's "polyvalent" anti-venin used for most kinds of rattlesnake. If a snake can't be identified a polyvalent antivenin is always the second choice.

Polyvalent antivenin is made by injecting a horse with 1/10th of a lethal dose for the horse. The injection is a mixture of venom types. The horse then acts as a stand-in for the future victim and develops the antitoxins he will require. For three months following the first injection the horse receives larger and larger doses about once a week until the dosage exceeds the lethal one several times over. Then the horse is partly bled, the red cells and other particles are filtered away from the liquid part—the part which contains the antitoxins—and the liquid serum is stored away. If the horse is given a booster shot it will continue to produce for some 6 to 7 years, totalling as much as 180 gallons (685 litres) of the naturally prepared antivenin.

Index

Gila monsters, 84–85, 186
puffers, 80–81
rattlesnakes, 72–79
scorpions, 81–83
stonefishes, 92–93
taipan, 93–95, 186
vampire bats, 97–100
Antiaris toxicaria, 18–20
antidotes, 5–6, 12, 22, 24, 36, 137, 154, 185–187
    activated charcoal, 68–70, 144, 145
    agate, 26
    "Ambrosia," 35
    antivenin, 11, 185–187
    Bezoar stones, 6, 27–29
    burnt toast, 144
    deafness, 6
    defined, 10–11
    diamonds, 25–26
    emeralds, 26
    Famous Pills, 42–43
    garlic juice, 10
    Hemodetoxifier, 70–71
    intoxication, 26
    kits, 144–145
    madstones, 31
    mandrake, 114
    Mithridaticum, 42
    "Nut Theriac," 35
    "polyvalent," 97, 187
    rattlesnakes, 79, 187
    snakebite, 10–11, 185–187
    snakestones, 31
    stonefish venom, 92–93
    stones, 24–31
    theriaca, 34
    unicorn horn, 38–39
    universal, commercial, 144
    universal, search for, 68–70
    warts, 6
    whiskey as, 10
    wine and hot pepper, 11
antimony, 45, 55, 70, 135
antipyrene, 70

antivenin, 11, 83, 186
appleseeds, 135
"Aqua Toffana," 52
Aristotle, 13, 38, 82, 130
Arizona scorpion (*Centruroides sculpturatus*), 82
arsenic, 45, 52, 55, 58–59, 70, 128–130, 167
arsenious oxide, *see* arsenic
Arunta of Australia, 16
asps, 85–89
Atropa belladonna, 48, 105, 112, 113, 117–118
atropine, 70, 110, 111
Attalus, 33
Australia, Poisons Control Division, 152–155
Avicenna, 37
Aztecs, 21, 129

Babylonia, 13
Bacchus, 26
bane berry, 179
barbasco plant, 21–22
barbiturates, 10, 70, 151, 159, 167
Barringtonia asiatica, 20
batrachotoxia, 102
bats, vampire, 97–100
B-D Hemodetoxifier, 70–71
belladonna (*Atropa belladonna*), 48, 105, 112, 113, 117–118
benzene, 167
benzine, 167
be-still tree, 124
Bezoar stones, 6, 27–29, 38
biological warfare, 12, 95
    "Dengue fever," 95
    "007 hardware," 7
    Q-fever, 95
bite of serpents, 26
black locust, 178
black widow spider (*Latrodectus mactans*), 89–91
bleeding heart, 175
blood red agate, 26
bloodroot, 178

blowguns, 7, 12, 17–18, 102, 103
Borgia, Cesare, 49–52
Borgia family, 12, 48–52
Borgia, Lucretia, 49, 51–52
Borgia, Rodrigo, 49
botulin bacterium (*Clostridium botulinum*), 66, 95–97
botulism, 95–96
    result of canning, 96–97
    symptoms, 96
bufagin, 102
Bufo (*Bufo marinus*), 101–103
Bufo marinus, 101–103
Bushmen of South Africa, 14–15
buttercups (*Ranunculus abortivus*), 182

camphor, 70, 114
cantharides, 70
carbon monoxide, 62–63, 131–133, 168
carbon tetrachloride, 168
castor bean (*Ricinus communis*), 105, 118–119, 120, 173
Celts, 13
Central American Indians, 24
Central Intelligence Agency (CIA), 7, 104
Centruroides sculpturatus, 82
Cephaelis ipecacuanha, 34, 70, 144, 145
Ch'an Su, 102
charcoal, as antidote, 68
Charles IX, 28–29
charms, 12, 22, 32
chemical analysis of poisons, 46, 54–55
chemical poisons, table, 166–170
chemicals and minerals, 128–139, 166–170
    antimony, 44, 55, 70, 135
    arsenic, 45, 52, 55, 58–59, 70, 128–130

secobarbital, 70
seco-brallobarbital, 159
"Secret Circle" of Venice, 46–47
"selective" poisoning, 18
semi-precious stones, 25
serpentine, 26
Set, 32
Shakespeare, William, 29, 86, 112
shamans, 23
shellfish, 104
silver, 45, 70
skunk cabbage, 181
snakebite, 31, 36, 185
    antidotes, 10–11, 26, 185–187
    cobra, 88–89
    poisonous vs. non-poisonous, 185
    rattlesnake, 72–79
snake charming, 86–87
snakes, 18, 185–187
    cobra, 85–89
    rattlesnake, 72–79
    kingsnake, 74, 75
    taipan, 93–95
snakestone, 27, 31
soaproot (*Chlorogalum pomeridianum*), 20
Socrates, 105–108
sorcerer's herb, *see* belladonna
"Spanish Fly," 55
spikenard, 34
spiders, 15, 89–91
    antivenin for bite, 186
    black widow, 89–91
    red back, 91
spring amanita, *see* death cup
Star of Bethlehem, 174
Stashynasky, Bogdon, 138–139
state of the victim, 67
Stoker, Bram, 98

stonefishes, 92–93
stone worship, 24–31
    agate, 25, 26
    amethyst, 25, 26
    bezoar stones, 25, 27–29
    diamonds, 25–26
    ruby, 25, 26
    serpentine, 26
    snakestone, 31
    toadstones, 25, 29–31
stramonium, 70, 110–111
strychnine, 9, 54, 68, 70, 127, 165
sulphonamides, 70
sulphur, 37
sweet pea, 175
Switzerland, Poison Information Center, 156–157
syrup of ipecac, 144, 145, 148, 163

Tahitians, 20
taipan (*Oxyuranus scutellatus*), 93–95
talismans, 6, 12, 22, 23–24
tetanus, 185
tetraodontidae, 80
tetrodoxin, 80, 102
theriaca, 34, 35, 36
    "Ambrosia," 35
    "Nut Theriac," 35
    Treacle (Theriaca of Venice), 42
thevetin, 124
tin, 70
toadstone, 27, 29–31
Toffana, 52
tolerance to poisons, 41–42, 129
    arsenic, 129
    Mithridates, 41–42
topaz, 27
topical medicines, 164
Topsell, Edward, 81–82

Toth, 33
Touery, P. F., 68, 69
toxicity, 56, 60
toxicology, 56–59
treatment of poisoning, 163–187
Turkish Stone, 27
turquoise, 27

unicorn horn, 38–39
United Kingdom, Poisons Information Centres, 150–152
United States, Poison Control Centers, 146–150
universal antidote, 68
upas tree (*Antiaris toxicaria*), 18–20

vampire bats (*Desmodus rotundus*), 97–100
venoms, 185–186
vomiting, 163, 164–183

water hemlock (*Cicuta maculatum*), 108, 181
whaling with poisons, 21
whiskey, as antidote, 10
wild cherries, 177
wine and hot pepper antidote, 11
wisteria, 105, 176
witchdoctors, 12–13
wolfsbane, 33, *see* aconite
women's bane, *see* aconite
wordless labels, 142–144
Worrell, Eric, 95

yellow jessamine, 177
yew, 105, 171, 177

Zoar, 26
Zopyros, 35